Massage Bible - A Beginners Guide To Western And Eastern Massage Therapy

Dr. Robertino Bedenian

Published by Dr. Robertino Bedenian, 2024.

While every precaution has been taken in the preparation of this book, the publisher assumes no responsibility for errors or omissions, or for damages resulting from the use of the information contained herein.

MASSAGE BIBLE - A BEGINNERS GUIDE TO WESTERN AND EASTERN MASSAGE THERAPY

First edition. January 13, 2024.

ISBN: 979-8224400157

Written by Dr. Robertino Bedenian.

Also by Dr. Robertino Bedenian

Fitness Over 60 For Women – How to Stay Fit And Healthy As You Age

Does Back Pain Go Away? 10 Answers To The Most Acute Back Pain Issues

Massage Bible - A Beginners Guide To Western And Eastern Massage Therapy

Going Vegan - How To Vegan Without Going Crazy

Chiropraktik - Was Steckt Eigentlich Dahinter?

Massagen: Ein Überblick Über Westliche Und Östliche Massagetechniken

Natuerlich Abnehmen, Schlank Und Endlich Fit Sein

P.S. Ich Liebe Dich: Wenn Liebe So Einfach Wäre

Was Tun Bei Rückenschmerzen, Bandscheibenvorfall Und Ischiasschmerzen: 10 Antworten Zu Den Häufigsten Fragen Bei Rückenschmerzen

Was Tun Gegen Schlafapnoe, Schlafstörungen Und Schnarchen

Self-Help Books for Women

Diabetes How to Help: Everything You Need to Know About Diabetes Type 1 and Type 2

Diet and Workout Planner: How to Stay Healthy and Get Fit for Life

Everything I Know About Love

The Sleep Easy Solution Book: How to Stop Sleep Apnea, Snoring, and Sleep Disorders

Your Super Gut Feeling Restored – How to Restore Your Life Energy and Overall Health from The Inside Out

Watch for more at https://booksummarypublishing.com.

Table of Contents

Massage Bible – A Beginners Guide to Western and Eastern Massage Therapy

Dr. Robertino Bedenian

THANK YOU!

First, I want to thank you for purchasing this book. My sincere desire is that this book offers great value to the reader in terms of understanding the world of massage therapy. It is written having entirely the patient in mind, who wishes to have a broad and a genuine understanding about what massage therapy is actually about. The purpose of this book is to give solid answers to those who take massage therapy into serious consideration as an alternative way of treatment to restore health in almost any part of the body. Due to my intensive research, I found out that several issues are addressed time and again when it comes to massage therapy. This book is intended to answer a wide range of questions patients might have or will have once they start engaging in massage therapy. After carefully reading this book, anyone should be able to have a very distinguished understanding of massage therapy. Furthermore, he or she will be able to form an unbiased opinion about this alternative way of treatment.

INTRODUCTION: MASSAGE THERAPY VERSUS CHIROPRACTIC CARE

Is there any connection between chiropractic care and massage therapy? Or is massage therapy just to be considered as another alternative way of treatment. Indeed, both are alternative ways of treatment, and both are related to each other. If you combine both methods in your efforts to stay or become healthy again, you will be amazed about the outcome.

If you are anything like me, you probably prefer staying away from providers of conventional Western medicine as much as possible, and I cannot say that I blame you. Although I have full medical coverage for that "you never know when you might need it" time of my life, I have not seen any of my Blue Cross doctors in well over fifteen years. And, honestly, I hope to continue not seeing them for the rest of my life. Please do not misunderstand me and think that I am some sort of superhuman creature who never gets ill. I do have my weak moments of pain and sniffles just like everyone else, or at least everyone else who takes good care of him or herself. So, when my body seems to need a boost, I visit one of my two favorite practitioners of alternative medicine: My massage therapist or my chiropractor.

I know that it all sounds very simple, but it is, in fact, somewhat challenging at times, because I do not always know which one of these wonderful professionals to seek out. So, I often first opt to visit my chiropractor for a good therapeutic session of adjusting and aligning my skeletal structure and then, as a bonus to me and body, I also make an appointment with my massage therapist for some hefty digging and rubbing. Between the two of them, I come out feeling like a million bucks although my finances are sadly depleted. I figure that we, my body and I, are worth it. Hopefully, this is or will be your attitude as well after you have read the second part of this book.

Now, you might ask, and rightfully so, "What is the difference between massage therapy and chiropractic therapy?" Well, let me explain to you:

Chiropractic Therapy

- For the most part, chiropractic therapy focuses on the *hard* tissues, such as the spine and other joints for adjusting and realignment.

- Chiropractors have some training in massage techniques, but that is never their priority.

- Chiropractors are authorized to make a medical diagnosis, order x-rays or blood works.

- Chiropractors cannot prescribe conventional medications, but they can sell supplements or homeopathic remedies.

- Chiropractors do not need medical referrals to perform their work.

Massage Therapy

- Massage therapists perform wonderful work on the *soft* body tissues such as the muscles, tendons, and ligaments, but they have not been trained nor are they licensed to adjusting the spine or any other joints.

- Massage therapists may not legally make a medical diagnosis, order x-rays, or do any blood work.

- Massage therapists are not permitted to dispense medications of Western medicine, but they can and do provide or recommend alternative herbal remedies.

- Massage Therapists do not require referrals from anyone to conduct their massage sessions.

A highly acclaimed national non-profit magazine conducted a study in which more than 34,000 participants in the United States were asked to rate which alternative treatments worked best for their two biggest health problems for the past two years. And the overwhelming majority voted just as I would have; for deep tissue massage therapy and chiropractic therapy in equal measures for such conditions as back pain, osteoarthritis, rheumatoid arthritis, fibromyalgia, respiratory problems, high blood pressure, high cholesterol, depression, insomnia, and prostate problems.

Of course, as far as alternative medicine is concerned, one should not discount acupuncture and reflexology for they are beneficial in their very special ways, too. We will delve into these methods of treatment among many others in chapters four and five. However, let us start by tracing back to the beginnings and roots of massage therapy.

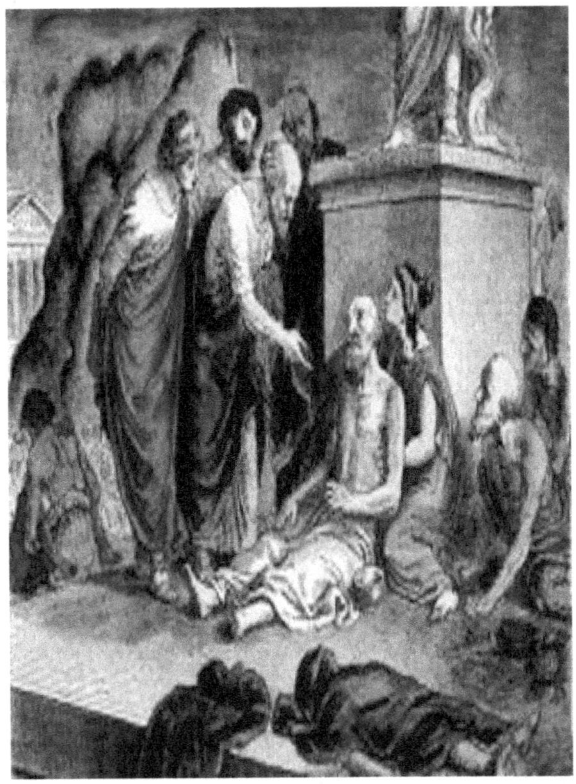

Hippocrates recommended massage to his pupils (source: http://www.planet-wissen.de)

1

THE HISTORICAL ROOTS OF MASSAGE THERAPY

The history of massage goes back into the ancient past. There are references of it among the records – written and oral - of many different civilizations.

The Chinese, the Greeks, the Romans, the Egyptians, and the Hindus all provide indications of a form of massage in place as adjutant to or an integral part of medical treatment. Egyptian tomb paintings depict people receiving a massage. Around 3000 BC, the Chinese made it part of a general fitness and health program.

The most well-known of these references to the use of massage during this period is the Huang Ti Nei Ching Su Wen or *The Yellow Emperor's Classic of Internal Medicine* (ca. 2,700 B.C.). It notes: "When the body is frequently startled and frightened, the circulation in the veins and arteries ceases, and disease arises from numbness and the lack of sensation. To cure this one uses massage and medicines prepared from the lees of wine." The book recommends the following approach:

"breathing exercises, massage of skin and flesh, and exercises of hands and feet" as the appropriate treatment for complete paralysis, chills, and fever."

In 1800 BC, Hindu writings indicated massage was part of a system of treatment involving such things as weight loss, combating fatigue, and aiding sleep. The Hindus writings indicate massage was also a tool in relaxation. We know more, however, about the use of massage therapy in Classical Greece. However, before focusing on massage therapy from ancient times until today let us take a more general look at this way of treatment.

OVERVIEW

Massage is rapidly growing in popularity. In the past ten years, the need for qualified massage therapists has increased substantially. It is not any longer the sole domain of massage parlors or wealthy spas. Now, you can find massage as part of an integrated medical system of treatment. You can see it in ICUs ("intensive care units") for babies, children, and elderly people. Massage is part of our care and in-house therapy as well as medical management for people with HIV-AIDS and cancer.

Nowadays, massage forms a small but significant part of many different types of health care facilities. Hospices, health care centers, and various types of medical and therapeutic clinics include some form of massage as part of a recognized form of treatment. In the sporting arena, massage is also a prominent fixture, making its appearance at the Olympics. Massage is also an accepted part of athletic training at all levels of the sport.

Yet, what exactly is massage? There is no simple single definition. The term has varied somewhat over time. In 1886, for example, *Thomas's Medical Dictionary of 1886* simply stated:

"Massage", from the Greek, meaning to knead signifying the act of shampooing."

A few years later, the definition became a little more involved. In *A Text-book of Mechano-Therapy* (1904), Doctor Axel V. Grafstrom declared,

"By massage, we understand a series of passive movements on the patient's body, performed by the operator to aid nature to restore health. These passive movements are friction, kneading, percussion, stretching, pressure, vibration, and stroking."

The definition for much of the 20th century continued in this fashion. A standard dictionary from the 1970s defines massage as a "manual or mechanic manipulation of parts of the body as through rubbing, kneading, slapping or the like, used to promote circulation, relax muscles, etc."

Online, the Encarta Dictionary defines massage as

"a treatment that involves rubbing or kneading the muscles, either for medical or therapeutic purposes or simply as an aid to relaxation."

There are other ways to characterize it. Some separate massage according to method or type. Some see it as traditional, others look at it as modern. There are Western and Oriental or Asian versions.

Massage has many types. It is not a solitary definitive action or typology. Yet, you can provide some basic parameters and, therefore, set forth a basic definition. Essentially, massage is the use of touch given by one person to another. Using manual techniques based on an ancient and/or modern system of treatment, the practitioner kneads, rubs, strokes, and compresses or otherwise manipulates the flesh. At its most common, massage induces pleasure. At its most powerful, massage is a tool for removal or reduction of stress as well as for pain relief, injury rehabilitation, health improvement, increased awareness, and/or athletic preparedness or recovery.

Although still in some instances a "naughty" skill or art, massage has become what it was once in the antique past – a medical, emotional, and psychological treatment. When you abandon the pure pleasures of the flesh in implementing massage, you are entering the realm of massage therapy. Massage therapy is a *specific* application of massage. Its purpose is to help the client recover from illness and injury or, as in the case of sports massage therapy, act as a preventative measure.

As a curative, therapeutic, enabling or preventative form of medical treatment, massage therapy may act alone or become part of a system of treatment. It may complement other traditional or alternative therapies such as chiropractic care as discussed in part I of this book. In doing so, it becomes part of a larger and often intricate approach to healing referred to as CAM (Complementary and Alternative Medicine).

The following pages of this book will guide you through the field of massage therapy. It will examine its application during the period from ancient times until today, the purposes, benefits, training, types, and terminology. It will consider the various approaches and techniques they use. From aromatherapy massage to Trigger Point Massage, this book will consider and discuss massage therapy and all its aspects.

MASSAGE IN ANCIENT GREECE

The Greek word for massage was anatripsis. The Greeks recognized massage in helping battle problems of fatigue and muscle pain among soldiers. They found it to ease the pain and release tension during training. They also applied massage to athletes both pre and post tournaments. Herodicus was the first Greek physician to implement massage as a medical treatment. He claimed it helped to prolong life. In his practice, Herodicus used massage together with herbs and oils. His student, the "Father of Medicine," Hippocrates (460 – 380 B.C.), claimed massage improved the function of joints and increased muscle tone. He felt the best way to massage a person was towards the heart.

Hippocrates mentioned massage several times throughout his writings. His most quoted references are found in "On surgery" and "On articulations." In the former, he states: "Anatripsis [massage or rubbing] can relax, brace, incarnate, and attenuate: hard anatripsis braces, soft anatripsis relaxes while much anatripsis attenuates and moderate rubbing thickens." In the latter, he writes: "The physician must be experienced in many things, but assuredly in rubbing (anatripsis), for things which have the same name have not always the same effects. For rubbing a joint that is too loose, and loosen a joint that is too rigid."

MASSAGE DURING THE ROMAN EMPIRE

Carrying on from the Greek implementation of massage were the Romans. Their word for massage was frictus translated as "a rubbing". Both Julius Caesar and Pliny were the recipients of massage therapy. Julius Caesar required massage to relieve neuralgia and headaches. Pliny sought relief for his asthma. Aulus Cornelius Celsus (ca 25BC – ca 50 A.D.), a Roman physician, utilized massage in his practice. His works De Medicina, denote the significance of massage. Of the eight-volume set, several volumes spend time discussing the use, methods, and typology of massage or rubbing. He claimed it healed paralysis. He also noted its use in helping with headaches. Galen, court physician to two Roman emperors, Marcus Aurelius and Septimus Severus, also discussed the uses and importance of rubbing in his medical publications.

MASSAGE FROM THE TIME OF THE MIDDLE AGES UNTIL TODAY

The following centuries after the fall of the Roman Empire were not kind to massage therapy or many other types of medical procedures. The Dark Ages or medieval times saw little advancement made in these areas. Furthermore, the application of massage required hands to touch flesh. This was too worldly and too sensual for the religious-minded and ruled the world during this period. The only exception to this approach was found in the Middle East and other non-European countries.

Of particular note in the development of massage in its medical sense was the man known in Europe as Avicenna (980-1037). This Persian physician, Ali al-Husayn Abd Allah Ibn Sinna, was a prolific author of both medical subjects and philosophy. He also wrote books of poetry and theology. Avicenna noted the object or purpose of massage was "to disperse the effete matters found in the muscles and not expelled by exercise."

In the Renaissance, massage began to become more acceptable again. This was specifically true for the royal households of that time. By the 16th century, Ambroise Paré (1510 – 1590), a French barber-surgeon, was using it as part of his medical practice. He became the official surgeon to four Valois kings: Henry II, Francis II, Charles IX, and Henry III. His work in these and other medical fields provided credibility to the art and science of massage.

The massage continued to sputter through the 16th and into the following century. Little, however, was undertaken to advance it in form or theory. In the 1700s, it made its greatest advancement, one that was to affect the formation of modern massage therapy. In this era, two men stand out prominently. They are Per Henrik Ling (1776-1839) and John Grosvenor (1742-1823).

THE 1800s TO 1900s

Per Henrik Ling, a Swedish-born doctor, educator, and poet established a gymnastics training program utilizing massage as a key component. The school he founded in 1813 was the Royal Gymnastics Central Institute in Stockholm. The method was medical gymnastics known as the Swedish Movement Cure. Ling borrowed much of his techniques of massage from the Turks. There are also aspects of Chinese, Egyptian, Greek, and Roman techniques involved. His new creation became known first as the Swedish Movement System or Swedish Gymnastic Movement System. It later gained the misnomer of Swedish Massage.

At the same time, Ling began work on his inclusion of massage as part of a healthy lifestyle. Grosvenor wrote and spoke about the use of massage as part of medical treatment. He felt the application of massage therapy produced positive healing effects in specific medical problems. He saw it relieving the difficulties of stiff joints and muscles. He said it was effective under such conditions as gout and rheumatism.

In the 19th century, a Dutchman and doctor, Johann Georg Mezger of Holland (1839-1909), created the final steps for the system developed by Ling. He provided the French names used in what is now Swedish Massage. Ling did not have specific terminology to describe the techniques he used. Mezger did. He applied French names to the specific strokes. As a result of the efforts of him and his students, Swedish Massage (Classic Massage in Sweden) has the following terminology: effleurage, petrissage, friction, and tapotement.

In the United States, two brothers, both physicians, introduced the practice of massage. They were George Henry Taylor (1821-1826) and Charles Fayette Taylor (1826-1899). Dr. S. Weir Mitchell in Philadelphia and Dr. Douglas Graham of Boston also provided support. Graham published several articles about the topic. He also published one of the earliest books about the topic in 1884. His book "Recent Developments in Massage" came out in 1893.

During the late 1800s and into the 1900s, further advancements ensured the survival of massage as a respectable medical treatment. John Harvey Kellogg (1852-1943) of Battle Creek Sanitarium used massage and hydrotherapy in his treatment. He published a treatise "The Art of Massage" in 1895. A year earlier, several women founded the Society of Trained Masseuses in Britain. It provided standards for study and the prerequisites for massage education.

20th CENTURY MASSAGE

Further developments and works on the subject of massage therapy followed. Sigmund Freud implemented massage in his treatment of hysteria. Sir William Bennett established a department of massage at St. George's Hospital in London, England in 1899. St. Thomas's Hospital in London was to retain a massage department until 1934.

In the early 20th century, massage therapy became part of a variety of treatments. Sir Robert Jones, Director of Special Military Surgery Hospital in London, encouraged the use of massage. He felt it helped to alleviate pain by improving circulation, reduced incidences of edema, and promoted the healthy sustenance of tissues. By the end of World War I, Kurre W. Ostrom published his book on Swedish Massage (1918).

Various types of systems of massage began to emerge during the early to the mid-20th century. Jiro Murai developed the Japanese form of Massage called Jin shin jyutsu and Mary Lino Burmeister introduced it to the American public in the 1960s. Janet Travel began to explore Trigger Point Massage in the 1950s, publishing her manual with David Simons in 1983. Ida Pauline Rolf (1896-1979) published 1963 her book on Structural Integration (SI), creating and promoting the massage method called Rolfing. Francis Tappan (1915-1999) published her work along with the pair of Gertrude Beard and Elizabeth Wood. Their work, the celebrated book, "Massage: Principles and Techniques" has become a classic textbook since its publication in 1964.

MASSAGE TODAY

Today, massage therapy is clearly distinguished from simple massage. Sensual massage still retains a high profile in the mind of the public, but it is no longer assumed a massage treatment is something covert. Massage therapy is truly coming into the respectability it deserves. It is returning to the position of esteem it once held.

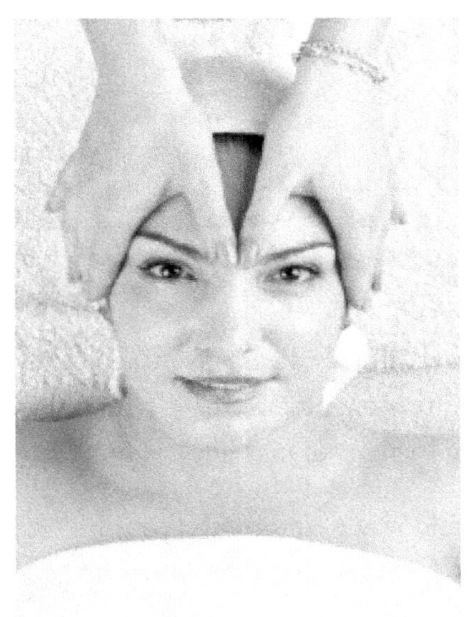

2

WHAT IS MASSAGE THERAPY ABOUT?

In chapter one, we have already been given a general idea of massage and its rising popularity. In this chapter, let us dig deeper into the characteristics, proper application, and benefits of massage therapy.

Massage therapy is a valid way of improving your life. It is beneficial for you in so many different ways. It is a method that knows no gender, age, or race. Touch is an essential part of all our lives. No matter who we are we can benefit from the power of positive touching or therapeutic massage.

Massage therapy can influence the health of people of all ages in a positive fashion. Babies and seniors can benefit from massage therapy. The sense of touch is more than a sensation. It is greater than a mere laying-on of hands or casual stroke. Massage therapy is a means of maintaining and improving your health.

Massage therapy, depending upon the type, is either directed towards a specific injury or body part, e.g. sports massage, or is more general in its scope. The purpose can also vary according to the practitioner and the client. It may be a matter of maintenance or an issue of rehabilitation. Yet, overall, the purpose of massage therapy remains the same – to promote and maintain a healthy body balance.

The following are specific and basic purposes of massage therapy. They cover a variety of functions and intents:

1. Relax the body, e.g. tight muscles and tense joints

2. Remove stress and anxiety from your mind

3. Stimulate circulation of blood and lymph to help improve various physical operations of the body

4. Help the immune system function at its best

5. Abet recovery or rehabilitation time of ill or debilitated patients

6. Improve overall health

7. Reduce and/or relieve pain –chronic and otherwise

8. Remove stress

9. Create or reinstate homeostasis (optimum health)

WHAT ARE THE BENEFITS OF MASSAGE THERAPY?

Massage therapy produces a many different benefits for the body and the person who inhabits it. These are not New Age babblings. Research provides support for several of the claims. Admittedly, more scientific studies need to be undertaken to provide further data, but to date, university research and studies made by the National Institutes of Health provide some validity to support the following:

1. Regular massage can increase weight gain among infants exposed to the HIV-Aids virus.

2. Patients after abdominal surgery have a quicker recovery time if they receive regular massage.

3. People suffering from hypertension show a decrease in their blood pressure after massage therapy sessions.

4. Sufferers of migraine headaches have a decrease in pain with a massage treatment system in place.

Increasingly, research studies are beginning to support other benefits attributed to massage therapy. These include the following:

1. Improves digestion

2. Reduces or lowers blood pressure

3. Releases pain-killing chemicals – endorphins

4. Balances hormone action

5. Improves blood circulation

6. Increases lymph flow

7. Abets muscle relaxation

8. Increases the range of motion for muscles and increases the flexibility of joints by lessening tension and stiffness

9. Reduces instances of joint and musculature swelling

10. Helps muscles and joints, sprains and injuries heal faster

11. Reduces the chance and extent of scar tissue formation

12. Mitigates stress and anxiety

13. Reduces pregnancy tenderness and discomfort

14. Introduces essential oils into the skin

15.Reduces dependency on medicine by providing an alternative pain management system

HOW TO APPLY MASSAGE THERAPY

The massaging of the surface skin, muscles, or affected part has several diffuse and related impacts upon the functions of the overall body systems. By applying therapeutic massage techniques, the practitioner increases circulation away from a specific inflamed or affected area. This, in turn, decreases the strain and tension on the affected parts. The result is a decrease in pain.

At the same time, rubbing the affected part or parts assists in draining the excessive or excess fluid built up in the system or area. This also reduces the tension on the body part. The muscle or joint, therefore, also regains some of the lost mobility. While massage therapy cannot claim to increase muscle strength, it does stimulate weak and atrophied muscles and joints. This, in turn, helps to improve circulation and improves the range of movement.

By rubbing the skin, the practitioner also helps to release endorphins. Endorphins are the feel-good, pain-killing chemicals in the body. As massage releases the endorphins, the patient feels a decrease in pain. As a result, he or she can relax. They can get more sleep. Bodies heal best when the patient is relaxed and inactive. By inducing endorphins to act, massage therapy increases the ability of the body to heal itself.

Overall, massage affects the autonomic nervous system by soothing the nerve endings of the skin. In doing so, it helps to calm d the entire body. It also affects the lymphatic system. The lymph surrounds every cell in your body. The lymph is responsible for supplying nourishment. Lymph system also carries away waste products. When lymph returns to the heart, it brings with it the waste products, viruses, and bacteria from the cells through the lymphatic vessels. The system contains filters or lymph nodes. These purify the contents, so they can then return clean to the heart to start the process over again. Massage makes sure there are no knots or blockages to the process. Massage also stimulates the production and flow of lymph.

Many illnesses are emotional or result from stress. Heart disease is one medical problem, for example, directly linked to stress. Massage therapy soothes the body and the mind. In doing so, it relaxes the person. It, thus, reduces stress and removes or decreases the feelings of anxiety, worry and even depression.

WHEN TO APPLY MASSAGE THERAPY

There are many instances when you can use massage therapy as part of an overall Complementary and Alternative Treatment (CAM) system. These include the following:

1. Reduced peripheral circulation

2. Lymphatic congestion

3. Muscle spasms

4. Tension, e.g. headaches

5. Anxious states of mind

6. Flaccid musculature

7. Backache

Some practitioners also claim the following problems or medical issues benefit, either directly or indirectly, from massage therapy.

1. Allergies

2. Osteoarthritis or rheumatoid arthritis

3. Asthma

4. Bronchitis

5. Carpal Tunnel Syndrome

6. Depression

7. Digestive and gastrointestinal problems, including diarrhea and constipation

8. Insomnia

9. Myofascial pain

Before you decide whether to treat your illness, check with both a reputable and licensed massage therapist and your doctor. Make massage part of a compatible CAM system.

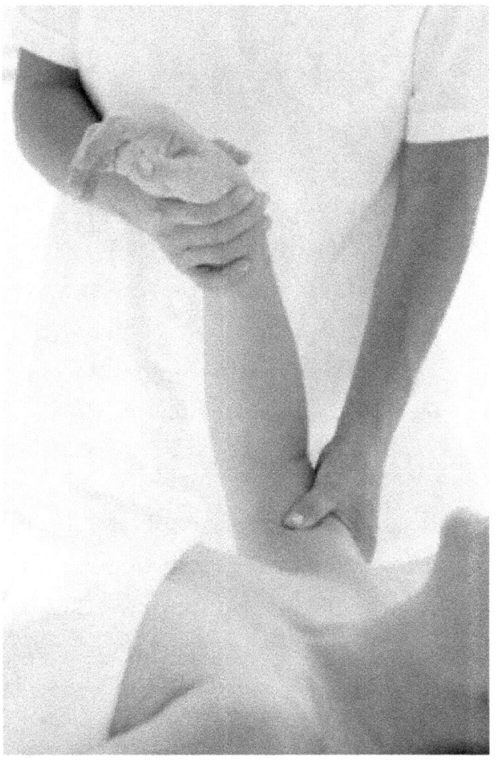

3

HOW TO BECOME A MASSAGE THERAPIST

If you wish to become a qualified massage therapist, you will need to go to school. There is, at present, no set path to pursue the career. Unfortunately, training requirements and educational qualifications vary from country to country throughout the world. The specifications for a massage therapist may even vary within a country. In England, Canada, and the United States, for example, differences continue to exist between provinces and states. It is up to the potential massage practitioner to ensure he or she receives the best possible education in the field.

There is no lack of good schools on massage therapy. There are many different college courses and training programs. The curriculum for each and the focus will vary. You may attend a course providing general information on a variety of massage techniques. You could also go to a college or school which concentrates on or promotes a specific type of massage therapy, such as Swedish, Sports, or Trigger-Point Massage.

CHOOSING THE RIGHT COURSE IS CRITICAL

In general, be sure to choose a course that offers you an extensive look at topics covering anatomy, kinesiology, and physiology. This will provide you with a solid grounding in basic body mechanics, physical makeup, and motor development. You will need to completely understand how the body works if you want to be effective in your career choice. Make sure you prepare yourself well in advance by taking courses in such sciences as biology during your high school years.

Besides courses in physiology and related topics, your selected massage school should offer a curriculum preparing you for the different types of techniques used in massage therapy. These should include a look at both Western and Asian methods. A basic overview of the types of massage should contain Swedish Massage and Traditional Chinese Massage. The two provide an excellent and comprehensive overview of the history and techniques of massage therapy you will require in your chosen field.

WORKSHOPS

Another way to eliminate what you like from what you have no interest in is to attend workshops. Many local colleges, ongoing education programs, and community centers offer special-interest courses. These frequently include massage instruction. Attend one or more of these to see if you have the personality, talent, and intent for becoming a massage therapist.

PRACTICE VERSUS THEORY

During the selection process, consider the number of practical versus theoretical courses offered by the schools. In the long run, it is the implementation of what you learn that will determine what type of massage therapist you will become. Therefore, it is essential to see whether your school has a focus.

- Does it concentrate on the theoretical aspect or the practical?

- Do you have sufficient sessions in applying what you learn?

- Is there an apprentice-type program where you can see and put what you learn into action?

BUSINESS SKILLS

When you determine your course of post-secondary education, look to see if the school offers courses in operating within the world of business. Such a curriculum will allow you to explore the options open to a massage therapist. These may include working in an office environment, alongside a chiropractor, out of your home, or in your office or shop. To help you make your decision, the ideal school will include financial courses. A reputable massage therapy school will provide you with information about such things as operating costs, location, financial options, and how to prepare a business plan. A good massage school will also not ignore the topic of ethics both in business and with your clients. You need to be aware of these issues if you wish to be successful and the best possible massage therapist for your clients.

Massage schools may also help you obtain gainful employment. They can provide you with guidance in selecting employment. Some schools offer job placement services for their graduates. They also continue to support their alumni with specific services to help them continue their learning. This may include post-graduate courses or workshops.

ACCREDITATION AND LICENSING

Choose your school with care. Check to see if the courses you are taking are not only pertinent but are accredited. Since some states require licenses to operate, be sure you select a school meeting with their approval. Be aware, your education is ongoing. In some places, maintaining a valid license involves continually updating your education and improving your skill through annual attendance at courses and workshops.

Be sure your school prepares you for the taking of any exams following your graduation. Some countries require you to take a specific examination before you can operate in their jurisdiction. In the United States, you may be required to take the Certified Examination for Therapeutic Massage and Bodywork (NCETMB). In Europe and the United Kingdom, there are different licensing organizations and exams. The licensing requirements may vary in different cities. This may lead to confusion. The Irish Massage Therapists Association (IMTA), for example, is trying to establish a national examination.

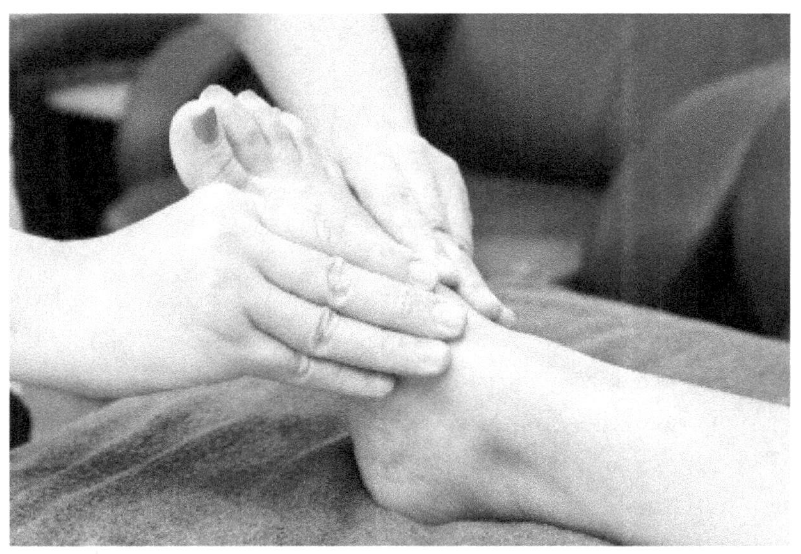

4

BASIC TYPES OF MASSAGE THERAPY

Massage therapy initially separates into two basic types: Eastern and Western. The former type is also referred to as Chinese, Japanese or Asian. While the two formats have commonalities, there are also differences. This is not simply a question of origin. It is a matter of philosophy. Western massage traditionally treats the body as a physical entity. It bases its approach on western ideals and understanding of medicine. Eastern or Asian massage looks at the body as part of a whole. It considers the physical, emotional, and mental aspects of a human being as one interdependent entity.

Within the framework of Eastern and Western massage, you find two basic subdivisions. These are traditional and modern eclectic. Traditional massage therapy conforms to the original concepts. They remain staunchly Eastern or Western in their outlook and approach to treatment. Modern, eclectic massage therapy diverges. It can be Western massage techniques utilizing Eastern philosophy. It could also be Eastern techniques with a more Western approach to medical concepts. Modern eclectic massage therapy essentially offers a variation on the original theme. First, let us delve into Western massage therapy.

WESTERN MASSAGE THERAPY

The original version of Western massage therapy is, without a doubt, Swedish Massage. In fact, in Sweden and among many practitioners, Swedish Massage is known as Classic Massage. It is a massage therapy based entirely on a physical or medical approach. It is the physical body that is of importance. A massage therapist of these and other traditional forms of Western massage focuses on the anatomy as defined by Western medical research. These massage therapists work within a tradition that uses the current concepts of the scientific understanding and findings on the physical entity we call the body.

<u>Special forms of Western massage include</u>

- Sports Massage

- Medical Massage and

- Deep Tissue Massage.

The massage therapists of these types of massage focus only on the physical repair and maintenance of the body. However, there are also different approaches to Western massage therapy. These types of massages, including the Swedish Massage, and many others will be discussed in chapter five in detail.

OTHER TYPES OF WESTERN MASSAGE THERAPY

Western forms of massage therapy are both traditional and modern. While Sports Massage, Swedish Massage, Deep Tissue Massage are popular forms, they are not the only types of Western massage available. Indeed, there are many different variations of Western massage. Some are simple adaptations of the basic Swedish Massage. Others combine the traditional with a more modern approach. Some unite Eastern and Western elements to create a new entity. Among the many other types of Western massage therapy are the following:

- Rolfing

- Myofascial Release

- Kurashova Method

- Esalen Massage

- Medical Massage

- Reflexology

Let us take a more in-depth look at those types:

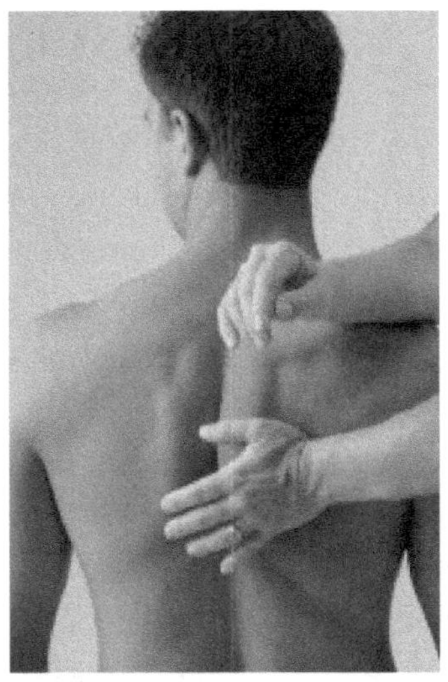

Rolfing (source: http://rolfingjourney.com)

A) ROLFING

Rolfing is the product of the work of Ida P. Rolf (1896-1979). The technique is officially the Rolfing Method of Structural Integration. It believes the body becomes worn d and shifts within the myofascial system (connective tissue). Using elbows, fingers, and knuckles, a practitioner helps to align the misaligned body tissue and joints. This is accomplished after ten sessions. Once considered a painful experience, the methods have shifted and become gentler in their approach.

Ida Rolf practiced at the Esalen Institute in Big Sur, California, before establishing both her method and her school- the Rolf Institute. Esalen Massage, like Rolfing, is based on Swedish Massage. Its techniques are similar. Esalen massage therapy features the long strokes of Swedish Massage combining them with rocking movements and deep tissue massage. Esalen does so in what they refer to as a caring or nurturing environment. The environmental factor owes much to the sensory awareness approach of Charlotte Selver. Nevertheless, the focus is on physical wellness.

Rolfing is also related to Myofascial Release massage therapy. The Myofascial Release approach owes much to the work of John Barnes, a physical therapist. The focus here, like in Rolfing, is on the fascia. The fascia is the connective tissue found everywhere around the muscles and joints, surrounding the organs, and bones. To release tension and restore balance to the physical body, the practitioner massages the affected areas. Fingers, palms, forearms, and elbows are brought into play. The therapist uses long, gliding and smooth strokes to stretch and mobilize the fascia. Like Rolfing, Myofascial Release massage therapy may be incorporated into other types of massage therapy.

B) MEDICAL MASSAGE

Medical Massage is another adaptation of Swedish Massage. Medical Massage addresses only the issues of healing the physical body. Its approach and techniques tend to vary according to the needs of the patient and the directions/prescriptions of the physician. Medical Massage practitioners work together with other health professionals to restore health through treating injuries and addressing the issues of other illnesses. The most common types of massage address such things as deformities, tennis elbow, sciatica, knee pain, sprained ankles, and repetitive stress disorders. The technique is illness-specific.

The Kurashova Method of massage therapy has its origins in Russia. It is a known form of medical massage introduced to the United States by Zhenya Kurashova Wine. The practice consists of more than 100 strokes. Depending upon the condition requiring treatment, the practitioner uses deep or gentle strokes. In essence, this method of massage combines Medical and Sports Massage elements. It intends to treat physical dysfunctions and enhance athletic performances. It can also help clients relax or re-energize their bodies. It is truly Western in both its medical and philosophical approach.

C) REFLEXOLOGY

Reflexology is often considered an Eastern form of massage therapy. It claims to have predecessors in the wall paintings of Egypt and Chinese Acupuncture. Yet, its founders are both Americans. In the 19th century, Dr. William Fitzgerald developed a theory on the interconnection between specific points on the feet, pressure, and the impact on the body organs. He referred to ten zones on the feet that would influence health if pressed upon properly. This is very similar to the Chinese concepts of meridians or channels and acupressure.

Mrs. Eunice D. Ingham, an American masseuse, adopted Fitzgerald's ideas in the 1930s. She wrote a book "The Stories The Feet Can Tell" published in 1938. This spawned the massage now known as Reflexology. The intent is to restore physical health by pressing the points of the foot. Each foot (or hand) has specific ties to an organ or other significant part of the body. Direct pressure releases the pain and helps the healing process. Reflexology naturally finds itself in combination with other forms of Western and Eastern massage therapy. Aromatherapy, Shiatsu, Sports Massage, Chinese Massage Therapy (CMT), Yoga, and other practices may include Reflexology as a technique. In some ways, Reflexology provides the ideal example of West meeting East.

EASTERN MASSAGE THERAPY

The standard form of Eastern massage therapy is Chinese or Asian massage therapy. This can take many forms. The most standard is acupressure. Its approach is strictly based on the philosophical and medical concepts from the East. It perceives the healing of a body to be realized only with the involvement of the life force. This is the *Chi* or *Qi*, in Chinese, and the *Ki* in Japanese.

In Traditional Chinese or Japanese massage therapy, the practitioner works with the energy or life force to heal the body. It is all about balancing the energy within the body. It is also about creating and maintaining a physical, mental, and emotional balance. In the traditional form of Asian massage therapy, the therapist is striving to restore a balance among all aspects of the body. Moreover, he or she accomplishes this using a system based on a concept of meridians or pathways.

A blockage of any of the 12 meridians or 8 channels, according to acupressure theory, will cause many adverse effects such as disease and emotional trauma. By placing pressure on specific points, the practitioner clears the channels. This allows the free flow of energy. As a result, balance is restored, and health improves. Other traditional versions of Asian massage therapy include

- Amma (Japan)

- Tuina or Tui Na (China) and

- Thai Massage.

All these forms of Asian massage rely on the philosophical and medical approaches of the East. Tuina, for example, works with specific acupressure points to stimulate the joints and muscles. Techniques are traditional Chinese brushing, kneading, rolling, and pressing. Let us focus on these three other types of Asian massage more thoroughly.

OTHER TYPES OF EASTERN MASSAGE THERAPY

Asian or Eastern massage therapy is not restricted to the popular few listed above. There are many different types of Oriental, Asian or Eastern massage therapy. This includes both traditional forms and modern variations. As noted previously, within the general divisions were modern variations and hybrids. Some forms of massage therapy are new creations based on ancient traditions. Others are further developments of existing forms of massage therapy. In some East meets West with an interesting twist on traditional concepts.

The standard form of Eastern massage therapy is called Chinese Massage Therapy (CMT). In essence, this is a term embracing all forms of massage therapy falling into the category of traditional Chinese practices. CMT can refer to Acupressure, Amma, or Tui Na. In some instances, the term used is not CMT but Energy Work or Asian Massage Therapy. The latter is a more suitable term than CMT. It seems more appropriate to use Asian Massage Therapy (AMT) when you include types of massage from Japan and Thailand.

The most common form of AMT is Acupressure. It appears under many guises and with different variations in both traditional and modern types of AMT. Tui Na (Chinese) and Amma (Japanese) are traditional forms of acupressure. Both types predate the more popular Shiatsu. The techniques, however, are essentially the same. Amma or Anma combines pressure point techniques with stroking measures similar to those of Swedish Massage. It directs its healing properties towards the meridians and channels the energy along with these points. Amma utilizes the theory of the five elements as part of the process. Amma is probably based on the ancient practice of Tui Na.

Tui Na is the forerunner of both Amma and Shiatsu. The at least 2000-year-old practice encompasses acupressure but extends further to include various strokes. There is pressing but also kneading, waving, shaking, pressing, percussion, and manipulating of the body at pressure points between the joints and along the specific meridians. Tui Na may also use herbs as well as manual manipulation and acupressure in the treatment. Various schools are promoting and teaching Tui Na. Tui Na, like Shiatsu, is an accepted practice in Asian hospitals.

Thai Massage is also similar to Tui Na. However, the roots of Thai Massage are in both India and China. This is energy work, but it is more similar to ancient Hindu energy work. The pattern of meridians is more Indian than Chinese. The methods, however, are familiar to Tui Na practitioners. The pressure of the palms and fingers is applied to the points along the channels or meridians. This releases blockages along the routes. Thai Massage also utilizes various stretches of the body. The practitioner moves the body in certain ways to help energize the body and increase the range of movement. An adapted approach of Thai Massage is Thai Yoga Massage. This type of massage closely aligns the practices of Thai Massage techniques with those of Yoga. The life force in this instance is referred to by the Indian word of Prana.

Eastern massage therapy bases its practice on principles of medicine predating Western concepts. As a result, the approach is very disparate from most Western practices. It bases its concept on the belief in a life force traveling along specific body channels (12 meridians and 8 other channels). If there is a disturbance in the flow of Chi/Qi (Ki) and a blockage, the person falls mentally, physically, or emotionally ill. It is then up to the practitioner to find the problem and restore the balance of the Chi. This is accomplished by pressing, kneading, pinching, squeezing, and percussing along the acupoints along the channels or the extraordinary acupoints, not on the channels. The practitioner does this to restore the balance of the Ki/Qi – the life or energy force. This is one reason why some refer to the practice of Eastern massage therapy as Energy Work.

The other prominent feature of all styles of Eastern massage therapy is the philosophical approach. This is a holistic treatment. It does not focus solely on the body. It intends to treat the whole person. It addresses the body-mind-soul aspects. All traditional forms do so, while modern variations may focus on one particular aspect.

ECLECTIC COMBINATIONS

Both Asian and Western massage practitioners follow their concept of physiology. There are, however, eclectic combinations. While some may base their origins in the past, there are revivals or recreations of the original. Falling into this mixed category are:

- Shiatsu

- Aromatherapy Massage

- Reiki

While some, such as Shiatsu and Reiki, base their approach on traditional Oriental massage therapy or medicine, they combine more modern approaches or updated practices. Aromatherapy Massage, for example, combines the use of aromatic oils with various massage techniques.

Yet, Eastern and Western, as well as all the subdivisions, all have the same goal – a healthy, happy human. How they achieve it is different. The techniques vary. The philosophy may be radically distinctive. However, the goal of making a person feel and act whole again remains true for all forms of massage therapy.

These newer or more modern types of Asian massage therapy, such as Aromatherapy Massage and Reiki, have a traditional basis but seem to many people very New Age. Aromatherapy Massage does have an ancient lineage. Its roots are located in India, Egypt, Babylon, Greece, and the Moorish Empire. Aromatherapy Massage relies on the power of scent, using essential oils extracted from plants with healing properties. The oils are sent into the air and rubbed upon the body. The method of massage can vary. The techniques may resemble more Swedish Massage than Tui Na. There is gliding, kneading, and friction rather than acupressure. The perception and applications, however, have more in common with Asian beliefs of healing.

Reiki is another form of modern traditional Eastern massage therapy. Practitioners say it has Tibetan origins. The variation today owes its origins to the work of Dr. Mikado Usui in the late 19th century. The Usui System of Natural Healing bases its healing therapy on the manipulation of energy. The word "Rei" refers to the universal aspect of healing while "Ki" is the word for the basic life force (Chinese Chi/Qi). Everyone possesses Ki and we replenish it when we eat, drink, breathe and go about our daily functions. If a person is unable to replenish the Ki, he or she becomes ill – emotionally, physically, or mentally. In Reiki, the channels conducting energy are frequently referred to as Chakras instead of meridians. The practitioner uses his or her hands to restore the energy. This involves an exchange between client and therapist. It does not mean the physical touching of the body. Reiki practitioners usually have no physical contact with the body of the recipient.

Reiki, Amma, Tuina, Aromatherapy, and Thai Massage are all types of Asian or Chinese Massage Therapy (CMT). They all have a single intent. They wish to restore the body, in all its aspects, to perfect health. To do so, a practitioner draws upon traditional concepts of the body. These may include various passageways where the energy force flows and pressure points. Using scents, pressure, and various other means, the therapist attempts to remove or replace energy, Qi (Chi), Ki, or the life force. The therapist may also remove blockages or obstructions to energy flow. In doing so, the practitioner hopes to reinstate the natural balance of the body and, thus, restore health to the body, mind, emotions, and soul.

5

SPECIAL TYPES OF MASSAGE THERAPY

According to the American Massage Therapy Association, there are five types of massage that are the most popular. These are Shiatsu, Sports Massage, Deep Tissue Massage, Trigger Point Massage, and Swedish Massage. All but Shiatsu represent a western tradition of massage treatment. All rely on specific techniques and intents to produce the best results possible for their clients. However, there are also other types of massages such as the Zen Massage, Balinese Massage, Hot Stone Massage, and Chair Massage. So, let us delve into these special types starting with Shiatsu.

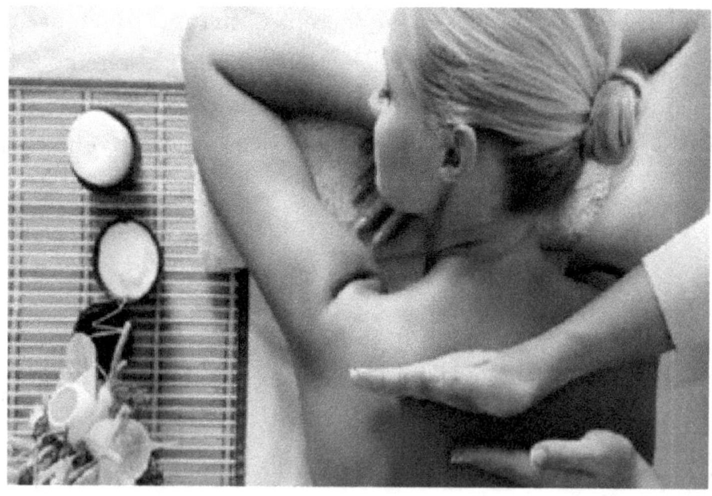

SHIATSU

Unlike the other four types of popular massage, Shiatsu looks to the East for its origins and traditions. Shiatsu is Japanese. It is often called a form of Chinese acupressure. Its name means "finger pressure." While considering some aspects of modern Asian medicine, it is principally traditional in its approach to human physiology. Moreover, it does focus on the overall concept of the interconnection of all parts of the human being: body, mind, spirit, emotion. The mind and body are an indivisible whole.

The technique of Shiatsu relies on knowing the interplay between the Yin and the Yang. A practitioner also has to be aware of the importance of the interconnection between the life force or Ki and the body. The Ki flows through the meridians or channels. Along these channels, there are tsubo or acupoints. If the Ki continues to flow without blockages, an excess, or a deficiency, then the body is healthy and balanced. If there is an excess (Jitsu) or lack of Ki (Kyo), there are pains, illnesses, and other health issues.

A Shiatsu practitioner is a giver. He or she applies pressure on the acupoints to balance the body energy and to promote good health. One technique is called tonification. It is a slow and gradual pressure. Applied to the Kyo Meridians, it helps increase the energy of the Kyo meridians. Another variation induces relaxation of the Jitsu. The basic techniques or strokes of Shiatsu to accomplish this are palm pressure, thumb pressure, finger pressure, and elbow pressure. Yin is soft touch and lingering pressure while Yang touch is invigorating and revitalizing.

The benefits of Shiatsu include bringing relief from the symptoms. It helps to ease chronic pain. A Shiatsu massage therapy treatment can stimulate the hormone system improving digestion and reproductive systems. Its major intent, however, is to restore the balance of the Ki to ensure the body is healthy.

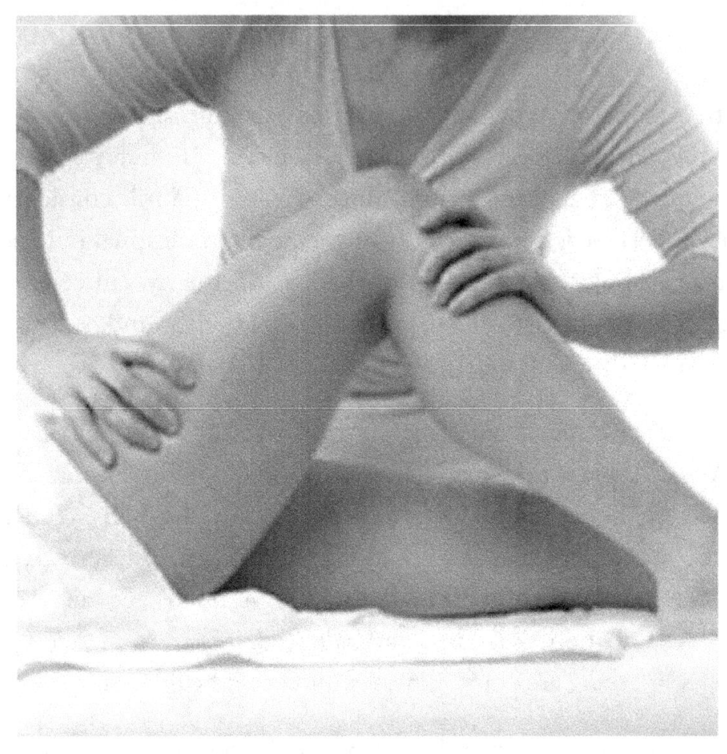

Sports Massage (source: http://www.medios-seminare.de)

SPORTS MASSAGE

Sports Massage is also a variation of Swedish Massage. It includes some aspects of Trigger Point Therapy. Sports Massage is a method of treating athletes. It is usually injury or athlete-specific in its application. Sports Massage emerged as a means to address the needs of athletes. This includes equine athletes.

<u>The techniques of Sports Massage include</u>

- Effleurage

- Petrissage

- Frictions.

In addition, there is compression and cross-fiber massage. Sports Massage Therapists may also utilize Deep Tissue Friction (DTF). DTF was introduced by an Orthopedic Surgeon, Dr. James Cryiax. It is similar to the friction used in Swedish Massage but goes deeper. It is usually applicable in situations of tendon damage and where there are micro-tears and problems to the joints and tendons.

Sports Massage also differs from Swedish Massage in another way. While the intent of both is to heal, Sports Massage is very specific in its intent and application. It is for athletes. Its popularity in sports has seen its inclusion in all major sporting events. These include the Olympic Games. Accordingly, Sports Massage is divided into three areas of application: maintenance, event, and rehabilitation.

Maintenance massage ensures the athlete can train harder and lessens the chance of injury. Event massage is divided into three components: pre, inter, and post. The former is a short-stimulating massage to invigorate the blood and relax the muscles needed to get the job done. The inter-event checks for any signs of damage and helps preparing for the next event. The post-event may be a one to two-hour massage intended to normalize the tissue of the athlete's body.

The most common type of sports massage, however, is rehabilitative. Its purpose is to ensure the athlete is restored to complete physical health as quickly as possible. It works on the affected areas to increase circulation, cut on healing time, and restore balance to the musculoskeletal system.

Sports Massage offers athletes at all ages and ranges benefits. It will reduce the possibility of injury, increase range of motion, and even the elasticity of muscles and decrease recovery time when illness strikes. The result of a regime of sports massage therapy is improved performance on the field.

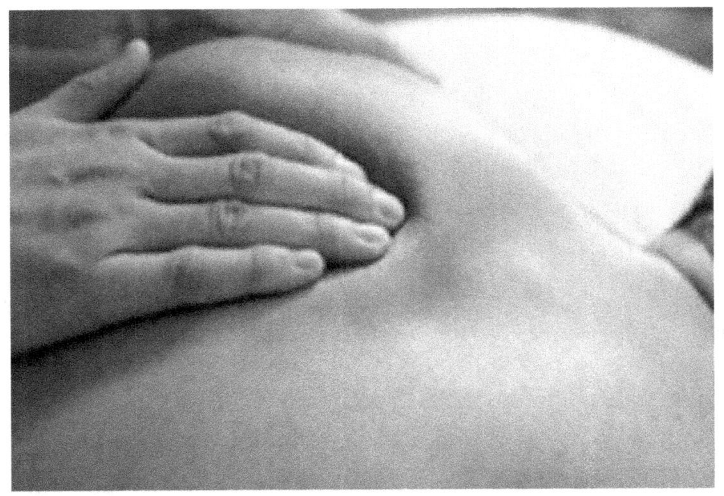

Deep Tissue Massage (source: http://www.körper-raum.de)

DEEP TISSUE MASSAGE THERAPY

Deep Tissue Massage Therapy is a direct descendent of Swedish Massage. In some instances, Deep Tissue Massage is a technique and not a specific type of therapy. It is utilized in different kinds of massage therapy. In Deep Tissue Massage, a practitioner can utilize several techniques to free the body from pain. It specifically targets the body's system of myofascial connective tissue. Here, the therapist may find adhesions.

Adhesions are tight, rigid, bands of tissue. They are usually present in ligaments, tendons, and muscles. In doing so, the adhesions block blood and lymph circulation. This causes pain, limited movement and often inflammation. The therapist using Deep Tissue Massage relies on slow strokes and finger pressure on these tight areas or adhesions. The approach requires depth in the pressure applied.

Like Sports Massage, Deep Tissue Massage is specific in its intent and focus. A practitioner will work to realign connective tissue and muscles at the deeper layers. In doing so, the therapist can address such health issues as low back problems, chronic pain, carpal tunnel syndrome, fibromyalgia, and restricted or limited movement of the muscles and joints.

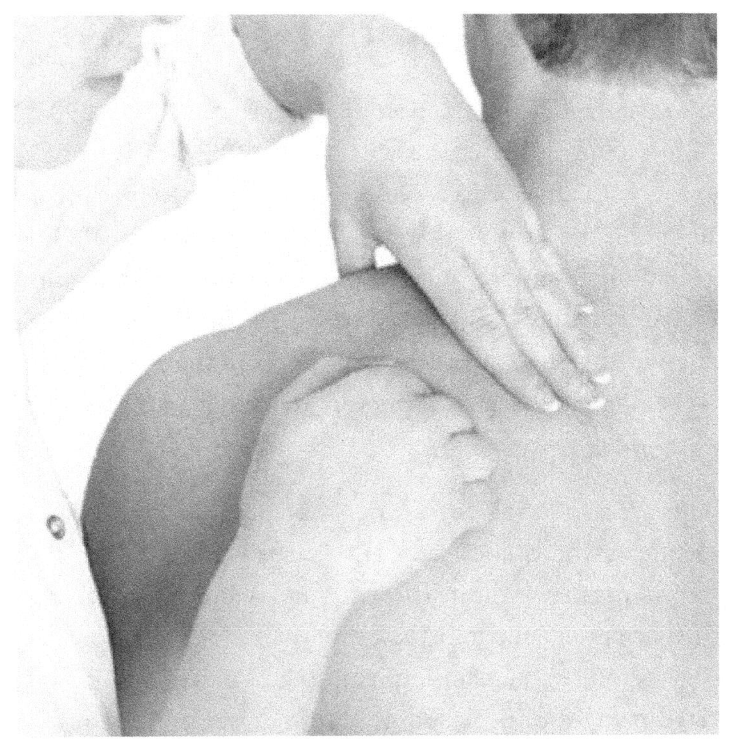

TRIGGER POINT MASSAGE

Trigger Point Massage is the creation of Janet Travell M.D. (1901-1997). As a former White House physician, she explored and, with David Simons, was responsible for the Bible on this variation of massage therapy: "Myofascial Pain and Dysfunction: The Trigger Point Manual" came out in 1983. It contains the basic techniques, purpose, and philosophy behind Trigger Point Massage. In essence, Trigger Point Massage believes the primary causal factor of pain and dysfunction is small, tender congested knots in the muscles. These are the "Trigger Points." Highly localized spots are responsible for pain in 75% of the cases.

Trigger points are responsible for a variety of pains, usually throbbing and dull aches. These include headaches, neck and jaw pain, lower back pain, and joint pain. Trigger points may indicate carpal tunnel syndrome. Earaches, dizziness, nausea, heartburn even colic in babies, sinus pain, or congestion can all be the result of trigger points. The defining symptom of a trigger point is something called referred pain. The trigger point is an indication of the problem which may not, itself, originate at the trigger point. Relieving tension and stress from the trigger point will, however, start the healing process and break the cycle of pain-spasm pain.

Trigger Point Massage recognizes three different types or regions of trigger points. There are central trigger points, satellite trigger points, and attachment trigger points. You may have an active or a latent trigger point. All affect the healthy functioning of the body. Pressure on the correct trigger point will relieve the pain and hasten the healing of the body. The method utilized by the practitioner is similar to Asian acupressure. Deep sustained finger pressure is applied to the trigger points to release them. As with Swedish Massage, Trigger Point Massage has also spawned variations and adaptations. Two specific versions are neuromuscular therapy and Bonnie Prudden Myotherapy.

SWEDISH MASSAGE

Swedish Massage or Classic Massage is the oldest of Western traditions. It dates back to the early attempts by Per Henrik Ling (1776-1839) to introduce a method of massage into sports education. In doing so, he integrated many different existent Eastern healing techniques into a Western system of anatomy, physiology, and blood circulation. Further development by Johann Georg Mezger of Holland (1839-1909) produced the current classical or traditional system of Swedish Massage. Mezger is particularly noted for the naming of the different strokes applied in Swedish Massage. These are Effleurage, Petrissage, Friction and Tapotement.

- Effleurage (touching lightly) is a smooth gliding stroke.

- Petrissage (kneading) is a kneading of the flesh.

- Friction (rubbing) is the deep, circular movements to the soft tissue.

- Tapotement (tapping) is the application of cupped hands, the fingers, or the edge of the hand in short, alternating taps on the body.

- In addition to these four original strokes, the massage therapist can use vibration (shaking).

In theory, Swedish Massage helps the body to relax while it improves circulation and increases the range of motion or movement of the muscles and joints. A practitioner uses this type of massage therapy to help an individual recover from stress and to prevent the onset of injury and stress-related illness. By relaxing the client, Swedish Massage reduces stress. This helps decrease stress-related illnesses. By improving the circulation, Swedish Massage decreases swelling around the injury and enhances lymphatic system production. As a result, healing speeds up and the reduction of swelling increases the mobility of the affected parts.

Swedish Massage is the traditional form of Western massage. Since its origins and with the increase of massage in popularity, massage practitioners have created variations. These include three on the most popular list. The offsprings of Swedish Massage include:

- Trigger Point Massage

- Sports Massage and

- Deep Tissue Massage

We have already discussed these three types above.

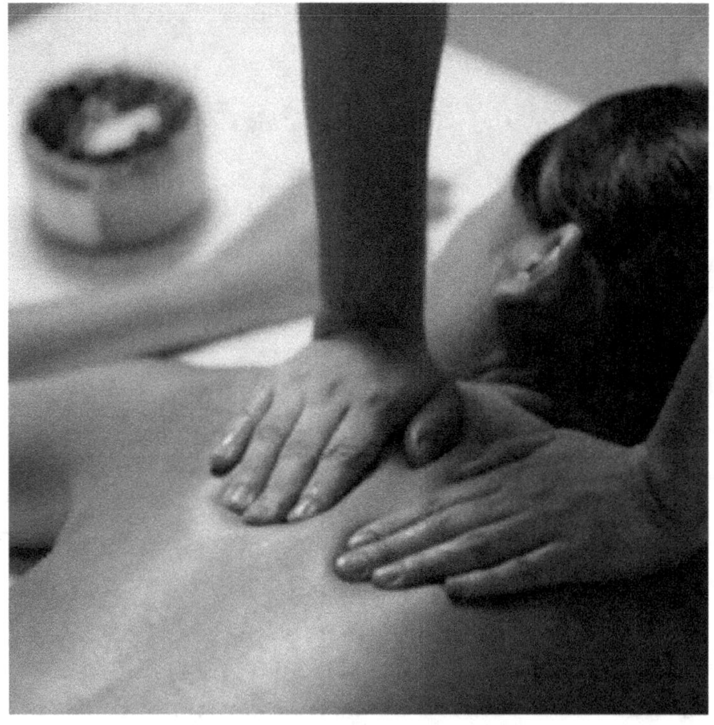

Zen Massage (source: http://zenbeauty.weebly.com)

ZEN MASSAGE

There are very many massage techniques in existence today; some of them stem from the far Eastern World of antiquity while others originated in the more recent years of the Western world. Although they were born of very different philosophical and cultural persuasions, each of these obtainable massage techniques provides some aspects of relaxation, but none does it as thoroughly as the one which was born in Austin, Texas, and christened as the Zen Massage. Zen, by the way, is an ancient Chinese discipline that means "meditation" and it focuses on the meditative portion of the *dharma practice* and the *experiential wisdom*, which is also called the *zazen* or the path of enlightenment. It, therefore, steers away from theoretical knowledge and theology.

By reaching into the very heart of hearts of every cell within the body, the Zen Massage epitomizes what utter and unequivocal calm, peace and a relaxed state of condition. Combining an assortment of highly sophisticated, time-tested and proven techniques, the Zen Massage affords its subjects a spontaneous soothing and an energy-balanced experience. The various features which are part and parcel of the entire therapeutic Zen Massage treatment are as follows:

The Heated Stones. This is a curative procedure that makes use of hot stones that are moved along the subject's muscles in smooth gliding motions and well-calculated pressure.

The Hot Towel Pore Cleanse. This purifying treatment involves the use of freshly steamed towels applied to the entire body. The heat of the towels opens the pores to cleanse and revitalize the outer skin (epidermis) while also reaching into the lower layers, the dermis, and the hypodermis.

The Bio-Mat. The Bio-Mat calms d and relaxes tight and sore muscles while it quiets and soothes irritated nerves. The Bio-Mat transports the subject into the realm of a complete state of well-being on the physical as well as on the psychological levels.

The Aromatherapy. Pure essential oils are used for this aromatherapy treatment to help the subject relax as stress is melted away and complete balance and wellness overcome him or her.

The Peppermint Bliss Foot Massage. The peppermint bliss foot massage soothes and softens tired and aching feet for a feeling of harmony and peace, which radiates from the tips of the toes to the crest of the head.

Zen Massage therapy is a non-invasive and natural massage treatment which has been clinically proven to be completely safe while being highly effective in relieving stress. This has also been proven to be the leading cause of countless physiological and mental health problems. Some of the most significant benefits that have been attributed to the effectiveness of Zen Massage therapy are:

- The lowering of high blood pressure which in medical terms is referred to as **hypertension** and has been often spoken about as the "silent killer."

- The improvement of REM **sleep**. The REM stands for rapid eye movement, and it is characterized by, you guessed it, rapid eye movements. It also includes rapid low voltage EEG, which is commonly spoken of as brain waves. On average, a healthy adult spends approximately 20 to 25 percent of a total night's sleep in the REM phase, and it is essential for good health.

- The decrease of **fatigue** of the body and the mind, which naturally leads to enhanced concentration and improved motor skills.

In conclusion, Zen Massage therapy helps its subjects to release their worries, unwind their bodies, relax their tensions, quiet their minds and ease their senses.

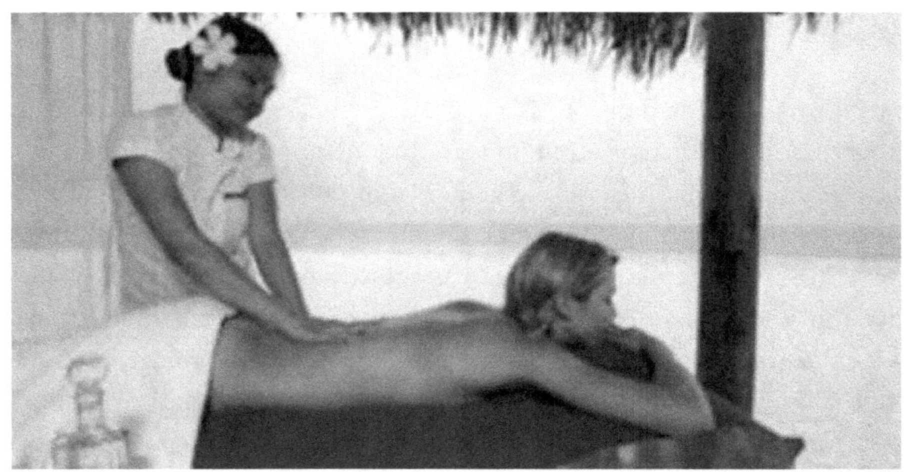

Balinese Massage (source: http://www.zankyou.de)

BALINESE MASSAGE

Having originated on the exotic island of Bali, Balinese massage is one of many ancient traditional massage techniques of Indonesia, which were carried from one generation to another as a method of curing a wide variety of complaints. The Balinese massage is extraordinarily unique as it brings together several alternative medicine practices such as massage therapy, acupressure, reflexology, and aromatherapy with the use of essential oils scented with striking aromas of jasmine, rose, sandalwood, coconut, cempaka, sandat, or frangipani into a single massage session. As it is true with most massage techniques, the Balinese massage strives to reach the ultimate state of relaxation throughout the body and the mind. What sets it apart is the Balinese believe that to attain that heightened state of relaxation, blood and oxygen must flow freely and only then will the *Ki* or energy flow without restraints as well.

Balinese massage therapy is performed on a conventional massage table or a soft mat on the floor. A great deal of attention is paid to the scented oils, which are generally applied at room temperature. For restorative purposes of an ailing or painful body part, warmed oil with an added mixture of lemongrass, cloves, or ginger is applied. Overall, the bouquet of fragrances used in the Balinese massage therapy is intended to induce relaxation, to promote indulgence of the body and to drive away nervousness and unhealthy tension.

To reach the deeper tissues of the muscles, the Balinese massage therapist alternately applies vigorous kneading, cross fiber mobilization as well as skin rolling with gentle motions to every muscle of the body. To enhance results with long-lasting effects, robust acupressure movements, such as hardy press points and strong palm pressure, are generously applied in addition to the prevailing massage techniques, such as sliding, long and short exploration, and manipulating.

Balinese massage therapy is far from being gentle or delicate, and it is, therefore, time and time again compared to *Ayurveda*, an Indian holistic medicinal method, which is considered by most as being extremely intense. And it is due to the inherent intensity of the Balinese massage that this therapy is so successful in reaching deep into tense and strained muscles to soothe and calm their spasms. Balinese massage therapy is quite frequently prescribed for sports injuries as well as for stiff and achy joints due to various injuries or ailments for easing migraines and other kinds of headaches, for relieving sleep deprivation and insomnia, for mitigating chronic and acute breathing maladies due to allergies and asthma, for boosting blood circulation and the lymphatic system, as well as for alleviating stress and easing anxiety and depression. In essence, the Balinese massage is a rigorous yet lavish therapeutic system that aims to bring the body and mind in full synchronization of optimal health, well-being, tranquillity, and spiritual renewal.

In preparation for a Balinese massage treatment, you should give yourself plenty of time to savour the entire experience and its afterglow. Under certain circumstances, your massage therapist may need to modify the treatment or the oils which are used, and you should, for that reason, provide him or her, if applicable, the following information:

- Are you pregnant or think you might be?

- Do you have any pains or stiffness in your joints or limbs?

- Did you have a recent injury or did you undergo surgery?

- Are you suffering from high or low blood pressure?

- Do you have any kind of heart problems or any other medical condition and are you going through some form of treatment.

Bali is just one island out of the 17,508 islands which comprise the Republic of Indonesia, a nation located in Southeast Asia and the world's largest archipelagic state. Many of the other Indonesian islands adopted their massage techniques, which are similar to the Balinese massage in their endeavor to heal the physical body and the spiritual mind. Yet, they are also distinct and bear their unique characteristics such as these:

- Sasak massage

- Lombok massage

- Urat massage

- Balinese Boreh. A paste of ground spices is used to relieve pain, and this massage technique was conceived by local rice farmers.

- Javanese Lulur Ritual. This is customarily executed on brides in preparation for their wedding day.

Have you decided to give the Balinese massage a try? Good choice! Relax, enjoy the process and come out smelling heavenly.

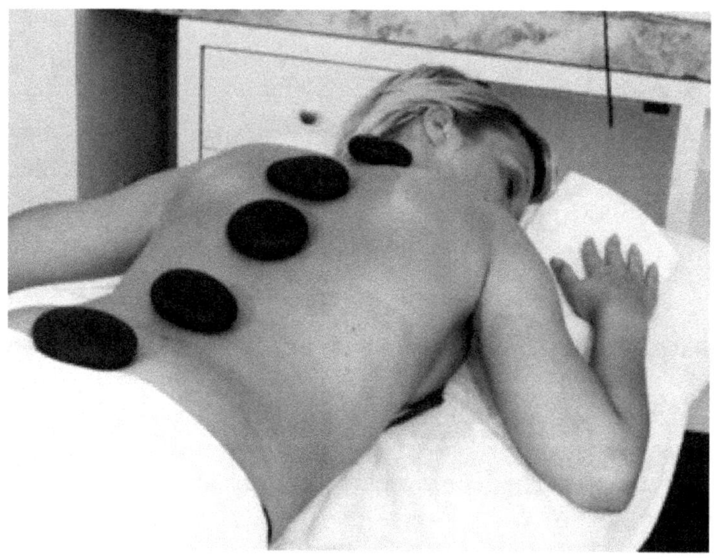

HOT STONE MASSAGE

The Hot Stone Massage is a therapeutic massage technique in which a heated stone is held by the massage therapist who uses it to apply the customary and traditional Swedish Massage strokes. Because they tend to absorb heat and retain it for extended periods, the stones which are used are usually smooth, black volcanic basalt rocks of various sizes and shapes. For the most part, these rocks are heated in water at 120 to 150 degrees Fahrenheit. Native Americans are known to also have used hot stones for medicinal purposes. However, those were heated by direct fire. This technique of fire-heated stones was restored by Mary Nelson, a native of Tucson, Arizona, and she trademarked it as LaStone Therapy.

Primarily, due to the effects of the heat from the stones, the Hot Stone Massage is profoundly calming and delightfully relaxing as it rapidly releases the tension out of every soft tissue, be it muscle, tendon, or ligament, which is included in this treatment while gentle and comforting peace washes over the client almost immediately. The hot stones are used throughout the entire session to massage, stroke, press, manipulate, and to knead the client's soft tissues. On occasion, heated stones are laid out to rest at strategic spots along the spine as well as in the palms of the client's hands and between the toes. This maneuver promotes the optimal flow of energy throughout the entire body. As soon as the stones cool down, the massage therapist will replace them with newly heated ones but areas that are inflamed, injured or swollen, will often be treated with cold stones instead of the hot ones.

To derive the most out of the Hot Stone Massage, clients are encouraged to:

- Indicate any discomforts such as those which might be created by stones, which are too hot, or by the massage therapist applying pressure with too much force, by the background music which may be too loud, by the room temperature which could be too hot or too cold and so on.

- Refrain from consuming a heavy meal and abstain from ingesting any amount of alcohol shortly before the session.

- Arrive in plenty of time to check in and to relax before the treatment.

- Take a sauna, a steam bath, or a hot tub before the session as it will relax and soften the muscles for better results from the entire treatment. If the hot tub was treated with chlorine, the clients are asked to take hot showers to rinse off the chemical.

- Remove all their clothing and be assured that they will remain completely covered with a towel. This will give the massage therapist better access and direct contact with the skin.

- Take slow, deep breaths throughout the session as it helps to relax the body and to release more toxins.

- To banish irrelevant thoughts from racing through their heads by concentrating on the feel of the therapist's movements over their bare skins.

- Get off the massage table after the session very slowly as dizziness may set in otherwise.

- Absorb the full results of the massage treatment by allowing some quiet time in a peaceful place.

- Drink extra water after the massage to flush out and wash away the toxins released during the treatment.

The Hot Stone Massage is beneficial in many ways as it promotes deep muscle and soft-tissue relaxation, eases stress, releases toxins, alleviates pain, improves circulation, and calms the mind. Quite appropriately, therefore, there is an impressive list of ailments, which are treated with Hot Stone massages and they are:

- Muscle aches and pains due to overuse, injury, or stress

- Back pain caused by injury, poor posture, or misuse

- Multiple Sclerosis (MS)

- Arthritis

- Fibromyalgia

- Stress, anxiety, nervousness, and depression

- Insomnia

- Any number of circulatory problems

The Hot Stone Massage requires specialized training. It involves more preparation time for disinfecting and heating the stones; the sessions are often somewhat longer than usual, and more time is spent cleaning up. As a consequence, the Hot Stone Massage tends to be more costly than any other conventional and basic Swedish Massage. However, it is worth it, and you are worthy of it!

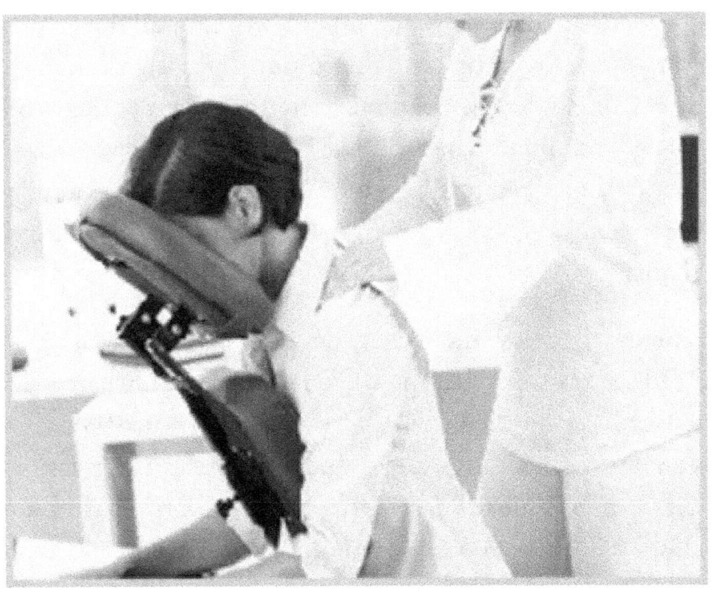

Chair Massage (source: http://www.massageausbildung-bns.de)

CHAIR MASSAGE

Massages in chairs or simply in sitting positions have always had their place among the most ancient and traditional massage techniques around the world. However, the contemporary Chair Massage as we know it today and as we occasionally refer to as the On-Site or Seated massage is a trend that began as recently as 1982. The Chair Massage was the brainchild of David Palmer, the director of the Amma Institute of Traditional Japanese Massage, who at that time was considered to be the "father" of Chair Massage. Mr. Palmer came to realize that, whether due to the high cost or the sensual intimacy of conventional table massages, or maybe the lack of sophistication on the part of the public or perhaps even due to the combination of the three in one proportion or another, there were too few people who sought such bodyworks services and, therefore, there was not enough work for all the graduates of his Institute. Mr. Palmer's entrepreneurial intuition and insightfulness led him to adopt a few existing old-time techniques and to renovate others to develop a modern massage technique, which could be performed anywhere as it required only brief periods, no need for the removal of clothing, and quite reasonably priced. Consequently, his Chair Massage became convenient, affordable, and non-threatening.

The first clients to enjoy the newly developed Chair Massage were the employees and customers of the Apple Computers outlets where David Palmer and his graduates set up their makeshift workstations in 1984. That venture lasted only about twelve months, and the demand at the time was not huge, but they afforded up to 350 Chair Massages each week. It proved to be a step in the right direction and a very good beginning. By 1986, a specially designed and structured chair to better accommodate Chair Massages went into production and, today, there are well over 100,000 such chairs in use within the United States as well as in many other nations around the world.

David Palmer realized that Chair Massage will be truly successful only with further development of this particular niche. That is why he offered to continue education seminars for training graduates of other massage schools. During the twelve months of 1986, he taught 24 Chair Massage seminars at 24 different locations in the United States as well as in Sweden and Norway. The concept of the Chair Massage was embraced with open arms when presented to the American Massage Therapy Association. As a consequence, by 1990 just about every massage school in the nation was teaching it.

The Chair Massage is not officially categorized as a therapy or a treatment but rather as a minimal relaxation technique. Whether that was a deliberate marketing ploy and clever salesmanship or not, it worked to attract people who would otherwise shy away from other kinds of massage therapies and treatments. For the most part, those who took the first step and braved the process of the Chair Massage would have become more open-minded about progressing and graduating into the "true" massage therapies.

Nowadays, Chair Massages are readily available in shopping malls, airport terminals, independent shops, franchises, hotel lounges, hospitals, gyms, spas, bus depots, train stations, supermarkets, community centers, eateries (particularly the new-age cafés), convention centers, beauty salons, barbershops, medical and dental offices, university campuses, corporate workplaces and even at street corners, public parks and city square throughout the United States, Europe, and the United Kingdom. The Chair Massage is estimated to be the fastest-growing and the most popular form of skilled touch, as professional massages are performed on the otherwise touch-deprived masses. It is David Palmer's greatest dream to see young children performing shoulder rubs among family members and friends as part of their regular daily routine. He expressed this dream like this: "When we reach that point, I will know that we have arrived at our goal of a world where touch is recognized as essential for the development and maintenance of healthy human beings."

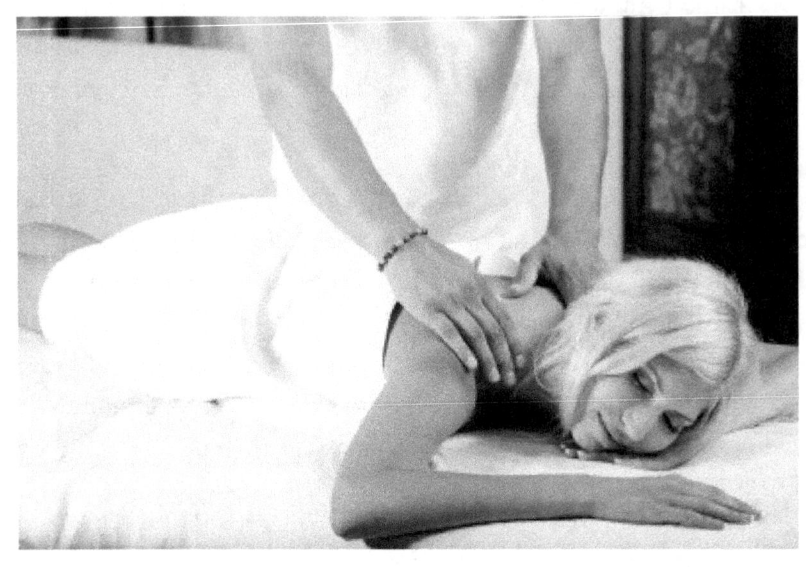

6

LOCAL MASSAGE THERAPY

Apart from the special types of massage therapies we have discussed in the previous chapter, there are also types of massages that focus on particular parts of the body, such as Facial Massage, Foot Massage, Hands and Arms Massage, and Head Massage. So, let us focus on these local massage techniques starting with the Facial Massage.

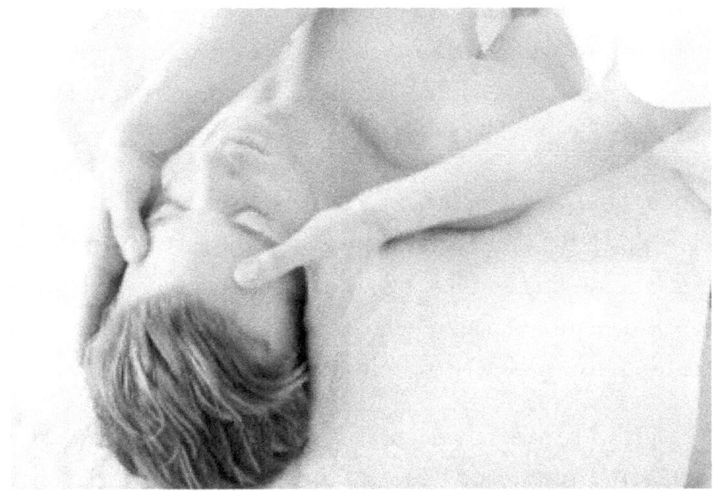

FACIAL MASSAGE

The oldest known Facial Massage in human history dates back to the third century BC where it was written about in an ancient Chinese medical text. Scientists have discovered many subsequent ancient medical records in archaeological digs conducted in Greece, Persia, Japan, and India. All these early-day writings have one thing in common; their Facial Massages were described in vivid details but always as part and parcel of total body massage therapies in which specific pressure points on areas of the face and neck were depressed sufficiently to loosen obstructions in the flow of the vital energy, which is also known as *Ki*. The standalone Facial Massage of the recent Western world was popularised in twentieth-century Europe before it was inducted into the North American world of cosmetic and beauty treatments. As a result, Facial Massage came to be regarded as the job for aestheticians, cosmetologists, and makeup artists rather than massage therapists.

In the cosmetic and beauty arena, Facial Massage is administered with the intent to slow down the natural aging process and to attain younger, healthier, and more vibrant looking and feeling facial skin. However, Facial Massage also has therapeutic benefits as it can relieve and mitigate stress, migraine headaches, premenstrual syndromes (PMS) as well as sinus congestion.

Despite their growing demand as entire massage sessions, Facial Massages are not precluded from total body massage treatments. Needless to say, Facial Massage treatments, which are performed the entire session, are much more comprehensive and include many elements, which are not included in Facial Massages that are part of full-body treatments. In both instances, though, gentle yet stimulating upward strokes are used in circular or semi-circular gliding movements. A typical and basic Facial Massage will include the following procedure and usually in that same specific order:

With the client comfortably reclining on his or her back on a treatment table and the professional seated close to the client's head, the face is thoroughly cleansed and wiped dry.

A lubricant such as a cream, a lotion, or oil is applied to the entire face and neck area. The Facial Massage will begin with repetitive rounded movements and will include every part of the face as well as the neck, ears, and scalp. Crucial pressure points will also be stimulated in the process.

The face, neck, and ears are cleansed of the lubricant used for the massage, and a facial moisturizer is applied.

Facial Massages may also include the removal of facial hair as well as the removal of blackheads and whiteheads, which will necessitate a moist steam treatment. These three elements will be included right after the massage session and before the application of the moisturizer. In addition, the entire process may be culminated with the application of full or partial makeup and sometimes even a hairdo.

The benefits of the Western-style Facial Massage are:

- Improvement of the facial skin and its muscle tone

- Relaxation of the facial and eye muscles

- Alleviation from tension headaches and general facial pain

- Relief from stress and anxiety

- The overall release of stress from the body and mind

Facial Massages are part of full-body treatments in Eastern therapies where pressure is applied to points on the face that correspond to various internal organs such as the stomach, the liver, and the gall bladder. With such different techniques, it is not surprising therefore that the benefits of the _Eastern_ Facial Massages are very different from those of the West:

- The stimulation of meridian points on the face

- Relief from eye strain and neck tension

- Correction of liver and fall bladder imbalances

- Recovery from nervous disorders of the stomach

- Release from premenstrual water retention

However, Facial Massages, Eastern or Western, are not recommended under the following circumstances:

- While clients are wearing contact lenses

- Open sores, boils, cuts, or recent scar tissues in the face or neck areas

- Inflamed, infected, or bruised skin of the face and neck

- Acne, psoriasis, or eczema, all of which can be worsened by the treatment.

Facial Massages are most often performed with bare hands that are lightly lubricated by oils or lotions to help them glide more smoothly over delicate facial skin. However, some mechanical devices may also be used instead of the hands or in addition to them. Best of all, in my opinion, Facial Massages can very easily and effectively be self- administered just about any time and anywhere, and countless resources on the Internet will instruct interested persons how to master the art.

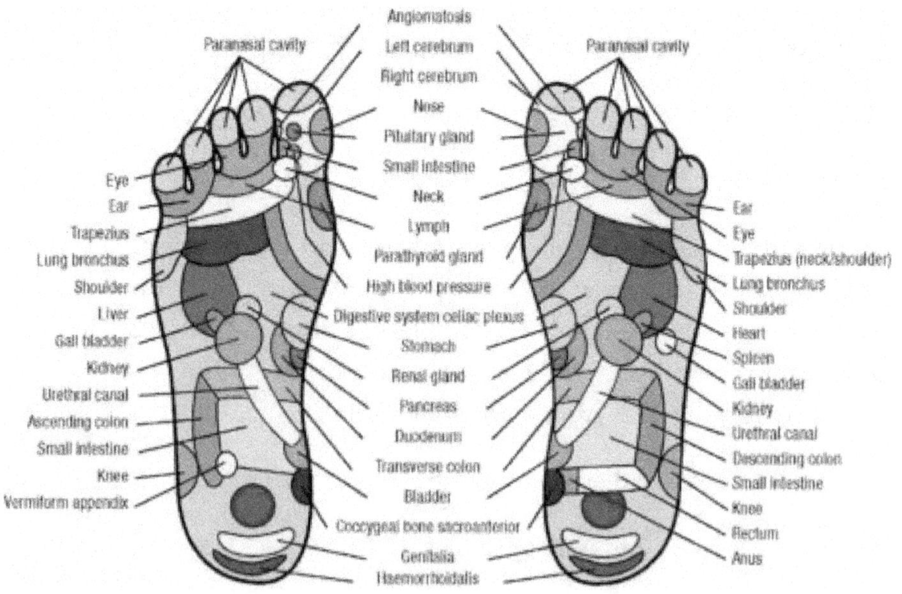

FOOT MASSAGE

About 2,500 years ago and during Lord Buddha's time in ancient India, a physician named Jivaka Komarabhacca developed a complex massage system which somehow ended up in Thailand where it was passed on by word of mouth from one generation to the next and is still practiced today in much the same way as it was so many centuries ago. When the Thai alphabet was developed under King Ramkamhaeng the Great, scholars began recording all aspects of Thai society, culture, and healing practices which, of course, included massage therapy. Unfortunately, future generations had little left as almost all was destroyed when Thailand's capital of Ayuthaya was captured by the Burmese invaders in 1776. All that remained of the recorded ancient traditions was that which, under the directives of King Rama III who wanted to preserve as much as possible, was engraved on the walls of Wat Poh, one of the most famous temples in Bangkok.

Based on the ancient teachings regarding massage therapies, many different kinds are practiced in modern-day Thailand. The Foot Massage is one of the most interesting of them since its principles are simple while its practice is quite a bit more complicated as the force, which is applied to the foot by the massaging hands, must be exceedingly accurate as it is directed toward particular nerves of the foot. The Thais believe that each part of the foot has a direct link to another remotely located part of the body such as a vital organ or a system. Therefore, applying pressure and massaging a certain area of the foot influences the soft tissues of that particular area of the foot as well as the other.

As a general rule, the Foot Massage is much more effective when the foot is bare in contrast to being cladded with socks or stockings. Several basic techniques are used by just about every Foot Massage therapist, and they are:

Sweeping and Rubbing. Most Foot Massages begin with bringing an increased supply of blood into the foot by rubbing its surface lightly but long enough to create the desired warmth and the rhythm of movement.

Thumb Walking. The thumbs are used to apply more direct and firm pressure to various parts of the foot as well as to loosen the tense tendons which run along the outside edge.

Toe Rotation. The toes are very sensitive and care should be taken when manipulating them by either rotating each toe individually or by gently pulling them upwards and outwards while squeezing gently.

Kneading. Kneading is accomplished by firmly but not harshly pressing and rotating the knuckles of a fisted hand back and forth across the sole, from its heel to its toes.

Cupping. This is a simple squeezing of the entire foot with an up and d motion of one hand while cupping it with the other.

<u>The Benefits Of A Good Foot Massage Are Many:</u>

- Firmly pressing and massaging the base of the fourth toe heals an ailing heart.

- Pressing and massaging the base of the second toe stimulates the lungs and the bronchial system for improved breathing.

- Pressing and rolling the area between the first and second thumb relieves headaches.

- Massaging between the third and fourth toe relaxes tired eyes and improves vision.

- Stretching and pulling the big toe alleviates pain caused by sinusitis.

- Rotating pressure at the ball of the foot will ease stomach ache and heal the kidneys, the bladder, and the entire excretory system.

- Applying pressure to the front of the heel delivers remedial effects to the male and female genital glands.

- Stretching the skin backward and forwards under both sides of the anklebone is therapeutic to the reproductive tracts of men and women.

- Pulling the knuckle of any toe backward along the instep eases spinal pain and improves posture.

- Holding the foot between two hands and rubbing the top of the foot between the first and second toe with one thumb while rubbing the top of the foot between the fourth and the fifth toe with the other, relieves the pain of the inner ear and the chest.

- Massaging the inner and outer edges of the foot is beneficial to the diaphragm.

- Pushing and massaging the soft spot beneath the anklebone reduces the pain from the sciatic nerve and stimulates the lymphatic system to cleanse the body of bacteria and toxins.

- Enfolding and rotating the toes achieves overall relaxation and a sense of well-being.

- With so much pressing, massaging, rolling, gyrating, pulling, stretching, and stroking; all the soft tissues of the foot itself become relaxed and invigorated.

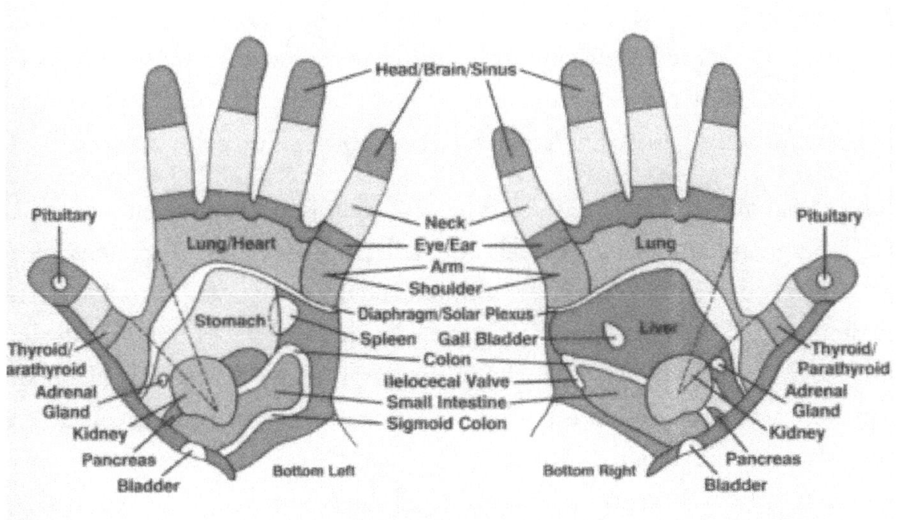

HANDS AND ARMS MASSAGE

From the moment we wake up until the moment we fall asleep, we all work with our hands, as they are our anatomical tools with which we perform the day-to-day tasks of living; the simple as well as the complex. Some of us use our hands to a greater extent than others in which case they may become painful, tense, and stiff. And since the hands are connected to the arms, chances are that the same hard work which applies to the hands also applies to the arms. As a consequence, the arms may suffer similar pains, tenseness, and stiffness. A mere five to ten-minute Hand and Arm Massage can work miracles in relieving all these unpleasant indications. However, a good Hand and Arm Massage also brings with it a whole battery of other health benefits.

Our hands and arms have scores of acupressure and reflexology points, which are correlated and linked to several vital internal organs (appendix, pancreas, gall bladder, kidneys, stomach, brain, spleen, heart, bladder, colon, intestines, lungs) and other remote parts of the body (sinuses, thyroid and parathyroid, hips, ovaries, testes, uterus, penis, prostate, spine, solar plexus, thymus, shoulders, knees, neck). A Hand and Arm Massage, therefore, does not only result in healing the hands and arms, but it also provides curative effects for such cases as poor blood circulation, arthritis, headaches, neck and shoulder pains, backache, digestive and reproductive problems, and so on and on.

Hand and Arm Massages are one of the easiest massages to perform on oneself and others, and they can be safely applied anywhere and to persons of all ages and genders; infants, young children, teens, adults, and senior citizens. Furthermore, Hand and Arm Massages are harmless to people who are dealing with most health issues, whether they are slight, moderate, or severe. Hand and Arm Massages provide instant relief from stress, anxiety, and nervousness as they relax the entire body. However, Hand and Arm Massages should never be performed on hands or arms that are affected by any kind of skin disease, infection, inflammation, swelling, bruises, cuts or recently broken bones, torn ligaments, ripped tendons, or surgeries. If and when oils or lotions are to be used during the Hand and Arm Massage therapy, an earnest verification regarding allergies should be made and any pressure applied must be tailored to the client's tolerance level to pain or discomfort.

A full Hand and Arm Massage should ideally begin with the biceps, the muscles in front of the upper arms, and those should be pressed and stroked upwards along the biceps from the elbows toward the shoulders and then back and forth across the tendons. When the biceps have had their thorough workout, the triceps, the muscles in the back of the upper arms, should be approached with similarly gentle pressing and stroking movement but this time moving backward from the armpits to the elbows. Moving on the arms by kneading the flesh, pressing the muscles, and stroke the tendons, the massage therapist should slowly make his or her way toward the hand that is awaiting its turn for a therapeutic workout. The hand portion of the Hand and Arm Massage treatment should begin by gently pulling each finger and thumb away from the palm while applying firm pressure to any painful or aching areas and then soothing them with moderate rubbing and rolling. The four fingers and the thumb should after that be pushed upwards as far as they will go without causing undue discomfort. The thumbs should be used to massage the palms of the hands by applying firm circular motions through the entire palm while intermittently stopping in various areas, particularly those which are sore, to apply steady and direct pressure for several seconds. For a soothing effect on the palms and in the closing of the Hand and Arm Massage therapy session, the thumbs should stroke the surface of the palms in an up and d movement.

A therapeutic Hand and Arm Massage can display love, appreciation, and devotion more explicitly than any other gift that anyone can think of. Just ask anyone who has ever been on the receiving or giving end of one.

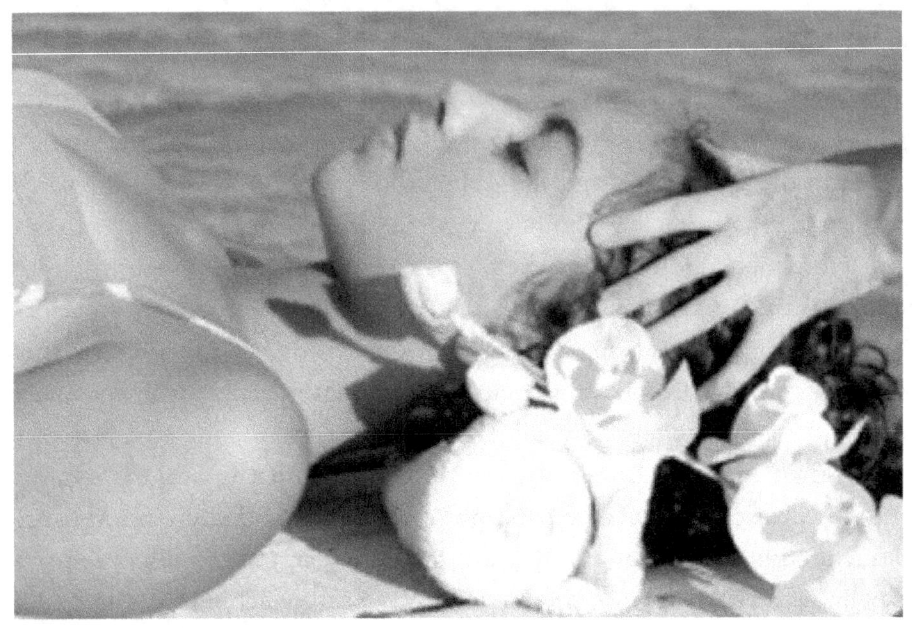

INDIAN HEAD MASSAGE

Its origins stem from an Indian remedial and grooming practice that had been and continues to be part of the Indian daily ritual for over 4,000 years. The ancient Indians believed that when energy channels become blocked and the flow of positive energy is obstructed, negative energy builds up and increasingly leads to a wide array of ailments and dysfunctions, such as stress, depression, poor sleeping habits, localized and remote pains, and aches, hampered and sluggish blood circulation, overall poor health, as well as loss of hair or even baldness. The main focus and intent of the Indian Head Massage, therefore, is to open up the blockages and to allow the positive energy to flow freely through the entire body and in the process to get rid of the amassed negative energy.

Indians in times of yore, young and old and mostly women but not exclusively, sat in large groups and massaged each other's heads. They began by applying a variety of nut and grain oils (coconut, almond, olive, or sesame) which were to nourish the hair and scalp while, at the same time, the massage promoted improved circulation. Today's modern Indians get their Head Massage treatments regularly in beauty salons and barbershops.

The Indian Head Massage was introduced into the Western world in the early years of the 1970s by Narendra Mehta, a native of Bombay, India, an osteopath, and a massage therapist. As countless techniques for the Indian Head Massage were passed d through the generations, Mr. Mehta developed his particular technique by integrating the head, neck, and shoulder massage into a single robust therapy that promotes and elevates the body to heightened states of physical, mental, and spiritual health and wellness. Mr. Mehta branded his comprehensive massage treatment as *Champissage. Champi* meaning "Head Massage" in Indian, and it is also, by the way, the origin of the English word "shampoo". With the help of Mr. Mehta's promotional campaign, *Champissage* rapidly gained popularity in Europe and elsewhere around the world. He summarizes his belief which echoes the belief of his ancestors by making the following statement out of his current home base in London: "Unfortunately, in the West, many people worry about their hair's health only when they start to lose it. Healthy hair should be promoted from childhood with the help of regular massage."

The body has seven *chakras,* which are centers that regulate the flow of energy all through the body. *Champissage* works on the top three energy centers or *chakras,* which are found on the head, the forehead, and the throat as it aims to bring the entire body into corrected alignment and proper balance. The effects are strong, silky, and shiny hair, relief from stress, restful sleep patterns, increased energy, and sharpened mental clarity.

The Indian Head Massage or the *Champissage* is performed in a quiet place where the client can sit comfortably on a chair, and the massage therapist can either stand or sit directly behind him or her. The sequence of the treatment is as follows:

The shoulders. Gently squeezing the trapezoid muscles at the base of the neck and moving outward toward the shoulders. This is repeated three times while slightly increasing the pressure.

The neck. The neck is massaged with small circular motions, beginning at the collarbone and ending at the hairline. This is repeated three times.

The sides of the neck are then stroked with a rolling motion beginning under the jawbone and ending at the shoulders. This is repeated three times.

Avoiding the vertebrae, the back of the neck is pressed with a gliding and rotating motion from the collar bone up to the hairline, and it is repeated five times.

The head. The head is moved slowly and gently forward and backward three times.

The entire area of the scalp is massaged with rolling gentle pressure four or five times and then the scalp is rubbed briskly without causing pain for a full minute.

The hair. Fingers are run through the hair from the forehead back three times.

<u>The temples</u>. The temples are worked with small circular massaging and pressing movements three times.

<u>The end</u>. Slowly, stroking the entire head area from the forehead to the back for a minute and progressively making the strokes lighter and lighter.

So far, we have been discussing all types of massage therapies, both Western and Eastern. Moreover, we have also been dealing with issues when applying massages. We have pointed out all the benefits of massage therapies. However, there is one question we have not tapped into, yet. Is massage therapy a safe treatment and thus applicable for everyone? Let us focus on this crucial question in the next chapter.

7

IS MASSAGE THERAPY FOR EVERYONE?

After we have been through all kinds of massage therapies one may wonder whether those promising massage techniques can be used by anyone. Are there any risks involved when applying those techniques or is massage therapy a risk-free way of treatment? Are there any side effects that should be taken into consideration? In this chapter, we will focus on the risks, if any, and whether there are groups of people who should not be exposed to this way of treatment. First of all, let us deal with the question if massage therapy is a safe way of treatment.

HOW SAFE IS MASSAGE THERAPY?

By and large, massage therapy that is performed by a properly schooled and well-experienced massage therapist who practices his or her art prudently and with due caution, is risk-free to its recipient's health and well-being. For that reason alone, if for no other, massage therapists must be selected very carefully as credentials and licenses are scrutinized meticulously, references are checked with diligence, and questions are asked relentlessly. Regardless of how it is phrased or worded, one question which must always be asked of a potential massage therapist is the following: "Which health conditions would you consider preclusive of massage therapy and why?" And the correct answer, whether stated in exactly those words or different ones, should be: "There are certain health conditions which must rule out massage therapy and those are ..." And he or she must name the following:

Cancer. Massage therapy comes in various forms, which affect the body differently. There are also many distinct types of cancers, and patients may be at different stages and receiving special treatments. In some cases, certain types of massage therapy may lead to life-threatening results while in other cases with another type of massage therapy the results may be extraordinarily beneficial. Because of such complexity, it is essential to consult with the medical provider who knows the particulars about the case in question before proceeding with a massage therapy of any kind.

The potential risks involved in performing massage therapy on cancer patients do not inevitably discard the entire concept of massage therapy. However, it means that extra caution must be practiced and, perhaps, moderate to extreme alteration of the treatment is in order. The health risks are the following:

Fractures of bones. Certain forms of cancer and their treatments weaken bones to the extent that they can easily break under pressure.

Bleeding. Many cancer patients tend to bleed easily. Deep Tissue Massage, for instance, can cause dangerous internal bleeding.

Spreading of cancerous tumors. There is an ongoing debate about the effects of massage therapy on tumors. Some claim that applying vigorous pressure to the area where the tumor is present will cause it to metastasis (break d and to spread or to increase its rate of growth). Others, however, deny that claim as unsubstantiated and untrue. It is best to play it safe and not massage the tumor region or its surrounding soft tissues.

Lymphedema (the build-up of lymph in soft tissue which leads to swelling of the limbs). Certain types of massage therapy in patients who have had their lymph nodes removed due to cancer may lead to lymphedema.

Flu-like symptoms. Patients who are going through chemotherapy can often develop symptoms, which look and feel like the flu after having been treated with certain types of massage therapy.

Pain. Cancer patients frequently suffer a great deal of pain, and most massage therapy techniques can result in some temporary pain immediately after the treatment. That may translate to added pain when too much of it is already present, and that can be quite unbearable.

Post-surgery. Shortly after surgery, the wound is still in the process of healing visually on the surface of the skin as well as internally. Applying pressure to the site may cause a series of risky health problems, such as reopening the incision, trigger internal and/or external bleeding or blood clotting, and so on.

Skin conditions. Areas where the skin is infected, inflamed, or covered with rashes or sores should not be massaged as it can lead to worsening of the condition.

Even when considering all the risks, that have been mentioned above, massage therapy can still be very beneficial to most people in most situations. Rather than discounting it completely due to specific concerns, I would advise consulting a physician.

MASSAGE THERAPY FOR ELDERLY PEOPLE

With the baby boomers aging and with the help of higher technology and greater innovations in medicine and geriatric science, life is not merely being prolonged but more and more senior citizens today have the opportunity to take advantage of more quality life than ever before. This translates into a generation of more senior citizens of more advanced ages living among us, and that is, in my opinion, a very good thing. National demographic studies tell us that nearly 40 million Americans are currently 65 years of age or older and over 2,000 more reach age 65 every single day. To accommodate the ever gr demand for massage therapy among senior citizens, many massage therapists are choosing to expand their expertise by studying the art of age-specific massage therapy, which is often referred to as senior's massage or geriatric massage.

For the most part, massage therapy for senior citizens is extremely beneficial and of utmost importance to relieve the aches, pains, stiffness, and the great number of health issues, which are so often associated with aging, such as inflammations in the joints, arthritis, skin discoloration, and other dermatological conditions, deteriorating muscles and bones, fading eyesight and loss of hearing, reduced appetite and therefore weight loss, poor blood circulation, sleep disorders, weakened mental capacity, tendonitis, bursitis, asthma, emphysema, high blood pressures, diminished functions of the internal vital organs such as the heart, the liver, the brain, the thyroid, the stomach, and the intestines and so much more. Most importantly, however, lonely and isolated, depressed, anxious, and fearful senior citizens derive pricelessly valuable benefits from the simple pleasure of the caressing human touch and the intimate companionship afforded to them during massage therapy sessions.

The Weaver's Tale Retreat Center in the State of Oregon conducted a two-year study examining the effects of massage therapy for senior citizens. They found that at least 50 percent of the elderly who were tested showed a reduction in their rates of breathing, an increase in their range of motion, an improvement of their postures, development of more body awareness, their skin took on healthier colors and their muscle tones were enhanced. The same study also showed that 100 percent of the senior citizens who were tested showed a dramatic improvement in their moods and their attitudes toward life in general.

Massage therapy for senior citizens does not differ in technique, but it does differ though, and it differs greatly in the application of that technique, whichever that technique may be. In other words, just about any of the different massage techniques can be used on senior citizens, but they must be modified enough to accommodate the facts that, very often, the skin of senior citizens has become thinner while growing much less pliable and, therefore, are much more easily breakable. Their bones are thinner and more brittle; their joints are stiffer with a reduced range of mobility. Their blood vessels are more prominent and closer to the surface of the skin and their overall health, vigor, and vitality have been degraded through the years. Taking all that into consideration, extra care must be taken when positioning them on the massage tables. They should never be expected to perform the same movements as younger adults, and wheelchair-bound or bedridden seniors should get their massage treatments while remaining seated on their chairs or reclining in their beds.

Most massages for senior citizens are limited to anywhere from thirty to forty-five minutes because the elderly seem to respond better to shortened sessions with greater frequency. Furthermore, greater time is usually spent on massaging their hands and feet than any other part of their bodies. That is especially true for those seniors who have lost the use of their hands and feet as massaging them will enhance their body awareness as well as increase sensations and blood circulation throughout.

We all need plenty of TLC (tender love and care), but senior citizens need and deserve quite a bit more of it. So, let us express our love and appreciation to them. Someday, we will be taking their place. And how grateful we will be when someone takes care of us in such a loving and tender way.

MASSAGE FOR YOUNG CHILDREN

Countless studies and pediatric research have shown that massage therapy is supremely beneficial for a wide variety of conditions in young children. These studies revealed that massage therapy for young children is a crucially important supplemental treatment to conventional medicine. However, these studies further showed that, in many cases, massage therapy on its own works better in relieving symptoms of many disturbing conditions than do medications and other standard procedures associated with Western medicine.

According to the National Institute of Arthritis and Musculoskeletal and Skin Diseases (NIAMA), more than twenty percent of all children, from newborns to toddlers and early school year children, are afflicted with eczema at some point in their young lives and roughly the same percentage is true for infants and young children suffering from traumatic burns. For that reason, the pain and suffering of trauma burns, and eczema are counted among the most common pediatric skin conditions in the United States. Most studies bring to light the following findings:

Young burn trauma patients, who were treated with massage therapy sessions for approximately thirty minutes before any kind of medical or nursing procedures, were more relaxed physically as well as mentally through the process and they, therefore, experienced less discomfort or pain.

It is important to stress here that the massage treatment was applied only to areas that were not affected by burns.

Young children suffering from eczema (also known as atopic dermatitis) who were given massage treatments before and while being treated with skin medications, such as emollients and ointments, exhibited less apprehension and were more willing to cooperate. In addition, the physical conditions of their skins dramatically improved as redness, scaling, excoriation, and pruritus subsided.

The therapy under these conditions ideally consists of two phases. In the first phase — to ensure smooth strokes during the massage treatment, the child's body is moisturized with a dermatitis medication. In the second phase — being very careful to avoid particularly sensitive areas of the body, a series of varied massage techniques is used on the child's face, chest, stomach, legs, and arms.

The Children's Mercy Hospital of Kansas City, Missouri, has been using massage therapy to alleviate chronic pain from headaches and migraines in young children and, in the process, also relieve their levels of anxiety and distress, lower their heart rates, improve their gastrointestinal systems, promote the release of endorphins and bring their entire bodies to a state of calmness. And all these positive effects seem to be immediate or nearly immediate.

Applying massage therapies to infants and young children is not at all a newly discovered concept as it has been a daily practice in the Eastern and African cultures for many generations. They understood that the first sense to develop in humans is the sense of touch that is essential to health and wellness. Massage treatments for the young members among ancient cultures served to heal, energize, calm and reinforce close bonding and the sense of trust and security.

Having been working zealously on the subject of massage for young children for the past ten or so years, Dr. Tiffany Field and her associates at the Touch Research Institute (TRI) in Miami, Florida, insist that "every child, no matter the age, should be massaged at bedtime regularly."

MASSAGE THERAPY FOR PREGNANT WOMEN

Who better deserves and needs good massage therapy than a mother to be? I cannot think of anyone, can you? Pregnancy is a very stressful time in a woman's life both on the physical level as well as on the emotional. By increasing the blood and lymph circulation, by lowering the heart rate, relaxing the body and easing the mind, massage therapy can be very beneficial on both levels as it relieves common symptoms of this delicate feminine condition: muscle cramps, spasms, and myofascial pain of the lower back, neck, shoulders, hips, and legs, the excess stress on weight-bearing joints, the swelling of the extremities (arms, hands, legs, and feet), sleep difficulties and the psychological turmoil (stress, anxiety, fear, and restlessness). Many independent studies have conclusively shown that the positively beneficial effects of massage therapy during pregnancy also benefit the growing child in the mother's womb as well as resulting in an easier labor and a less painful delivery.

What Is The Difference Between Pregnancy Massage And Any Other Massage? Well, there are several very important differences, which should not be overlooked. And due to those differences, therapists who perform massage therapy for pregnant women must be specially trained and certified accordingly. And they must always take those extra few precautionary measures:

- Pregnancy massage should not be performed until the first trimester of the pregnancy has been concluded because the increased blood circulation may lead to dizziness and a worsening of the existing morning sickness symptoms.

- Positioning of the pregnant woman is detrimental to her safety and the safety of the child she is carrying. If using a massage table for the pregnancy massage session, it must be a semi-reclining table. In case such an appropriate table is not available, the pregnant woman should lie on her side and switch sides in mid-session to make both her hips available for the massage treatment. A wide variety of pillows (body pillows, wedge pillows, and extra padding pillows) set in a few strategic places under the pregnant woman's body can greatly add to her comfort.

- Important safety measures: The pregnant woman must never lie directly on her belly and the flat, horizontal table with the hole for the belly must never be used as it inflicts too much stress on her lower back.

- Certain parts of the pregnant woman's body must never be massaged or pressed. These are both sides of the ankles as well as the webbing between the thumbs. The index fingers are pressure points that can induce early labor when exposed to sustained pressure.

For the great majority of the time, pregnancy massages are perfectly safe and much advised. However, under certain very specific conditions, pregnancy massages should not be attempted without consulting a medical specialist. Those conditions may be women who are at risk of pre-term labour and women with blood clots or related blood clotting disorders.

How Are Pregnancy Massages And Any Other Massages Similar To One Another? Every human being (pregnant or not, female or male, young or old, rich or poor) enjoys the touch of another human being as it conveys comfort, love, awareness, caring, security, and many other wonderful sensations. Pregnancy massage as well as any other kind of massage provides all that and more.

WHAT ABOUT SELF-MASSAGE?

Are you aware of having a personal massage therapist, actually two of them, available to you and ready to serve your wishes twenty-four hours a day and seven days a week all year round and charge you not a dime? And would you believe me when I tell you that these massage therapists are perfectly happy to provide you with therapeutic sessions anywhere you please (your bedroom or living room, your office or car, in a public park, or at the library), as frequently as you summon them and for the duration of your choosing? I am talking about your two hands. Yes, your two hands are perfectly capable of massaging away your stress, your tension, your stiffness and your pains while bringing forth an increase of blood circulation to invigorate and rejuvenate you with a fresh supply of oxygen into every cell in your body. Research shows that massage therapy, whether it is performed by a paid professional massage therapist or by your built-in and securely affix hands, also boosts your immune systems as the production of white blood cells is stimulated in the process as is your mental capacity.

Chances are that you probably perform self-massage therapy regularly without ever calling it that. Stroking your forehead in a spontaneous reaction to a headache, grabbing the back of your neck to squeeze aware aches and stiffness, scrubbing yourself d with a loofah sponge in the shower or bath, rubbing your sore feet after a long day or hard work are all forms of self-applied massage therapy. Congratulations! You are an experienced self-massage therapist, and you did not require formal training, a certification, or a license.

The following is a list of techniques you can safely apply to your body and promote overall wellness from the tip of your toes up to your head:

Upon Awaking And Upon Going To Sleep. Twice a day, morning and evening, treat yourself to a session of gentle punches. Always moving in an upward motion from bottom to top, begin with the legs, proceed to the arms, then the torso, the back, the head, and the face. This will beat out the tension, stress, and kinks in your muscles. Even more, it will improve your blood circulation and will strengthen your body.

A Treat After Dessert. Whether you have had a large meal or a small one, help your digestive process by rubbing your tummy in the same clockwise direction as your food travels through the systems. Therefore, use the palms of both your hands in a clockwise circular motion.

A Therapeutic Exercise Before And After For The More Athletic Type. Punch yourself before stretching, cardiovascular or strength exercises to get more blood flowing into your muscles. After exercising, rubbing your muscles in the direction of your heart will promote the elimination of metabolic waste as well as expedite the relaxation and recovery of your muscles.

Massage Your Hands And Feet. You may do this with or without lotion, but you should do it daily. Intertwine the fingers of both hands and rub the heels against each other in a circular motion. With one thumb, rub the entire palm of the other hand and then switch. Untwine your fingers and thoroughly kneading each hand, gently pull on each finger and finish by pinching the webbing between the thumb and the index finger of each hand.

Play Tennis Without A Racquet. To exorcise tension and stress, massage your feet by stepping on a tennis ball. A gulf ball will work just as well. From a standing position press one foot on top of the ball, apply as much weight as you can, and slowly move your foot around.

8

CONCLUSION

In recent years, massage therapy has shaken off its image of seedy massage parlors providing sexual services to clients. It has also abandoned the image of pampered rich people at spas or in exclusive health clubs. Today, massage therapy is for everyone. Many medical insurance plans even include massage therapy under basic coverage. It is truly coming of age.

Massage addresses medical issues, treats injuries, and helps people recover emotionally and physically. Sports Massage helps athletes maintain peak performance. Massage also helps sufferers escape chronic pain and new-born mothers avoid postpartum depression. More and more research is beginning to show the positive healing effects of massage therapy. It can alleviate various forms of medical problems and emotionally based health issues.

Massage is a wise career choice, although there are still issues concerning universal requirements for licensing and practicing. There are so many different options within the field. There is Asian Massage Therapy (AMT) with its emphasis on the holistic approach to healing through massage. There is also the physical philosophy of Swedish, Sports, and Medical Massage. In between these two types are the eclectic versions of massage therapy, including Reiki and Reflexology. These draw upon Western and/or Asian traditions to create a new entity.

Massage therapy is an alternative means to health. It is a different approach to help heal, repair, and transform the body. Together with chiropractic techniques, massage therapy provides an excellent form of both Complementary and Alternative Medicine (CAM) and holistic healing, including body, mind, and soul.

9

TERMINOLOGY

The following pages will help guide you through the world of massage therapy. They include basic terms and types of massage therapy. These include some forms not mentioned in or only referred to in the preceding chapters. The list is alphabetical in an attempt to facilitate the process.

Acupressure:

A method of Chinese Traditional Massage (CTM) involving the pressure of fingers and other body parts on specific central points along the Qi or Ki energy channels or meridians. Types of massage therapies using acupressure include Shiatsu.

Amma:

The traditional massage therapy from Japan. Amma or Anma precedes Shiatsu. Based on Chinese traditional forms, Amma uses acupressure, stroking, kneading, and percussion along the meridians.

Aromatherapy Massage:

Massage combining aromatic essential oils to awaken the senses and lead to healing.

Asian Massage Therapy:

The overall term for the various types of massage therapy with origins in the Eastern or Oriental forms. The focus in Asian Massage Therapy (AMT) is not solely on the physical body. The approach is holistic, including the soul, mind, emotions, and body as an integral part of the healing process. Asian Massage Therapy also relies on Oriental traditional concepts of medical and physical properties and anatomy of the body. As a result, there is a belief in the need for a practitioner to address the energy level or life force – the Ki, Qi, or Chi. By analyzing the energy flow through a system of Chakras, Channels, or Meridians, the practitioner knows where to press, knead or use other methods to stimulate or correct the energy flow through the body. Types of Asian Massage Therapy include Shiatsu, Amma, Tui Na, and Thai Massage.

Ayurveda:

A type of healing system based on the ancient Vedic writings of Indians. Deepak Chopra is a classic example of this form of healing. It includes massage therapy as one part of an integrated approach to healing.

Chakras:

Often defined as an aura, a Chakra is one of the seven centers of energy regulating the flow of energy between the body and mind concept. It is Indian in origin and often appears in the terminology of Reiki practitioners as well as New Age therapists.

Channels:

A channel is an invisible passageway for the flow of energy throughout the body. It is sometimes called a meridian. The channel concept is part of the overall Eastern or Asian approach to medicine.

Chi:

This is the Chinese word for energy or life force. It is responsible in traditional Chinese medicine for the health of the body, the mind, and emotions. It flows through various meridians throughout the body. If there is too much Chi, too little Chi, or a blockage of

Chi, the person will fall ill. Traditional practitioners work to restore balance to the Chi. In doing this, they will ensure the return to health. Chi is also Qi in Chinese. It is Ki in Japanese and Prana in Indian massage practices.

Connective Tissue Massage:

Developed in the 1930s in Germany, this form of massage therapy focuses on the layers of tissue between skin and muscle known as connective tissue. It proposes that massaging one area of the body will have positive effects on another.

Deep Tissue Massage:

This is both a specific form of massage and a technique used in other types of massage therapy. It involves deep manipulation of the myofascial connective tissue. Deep Tissue Massage owes much to both Swedish Massage and Structural Integration.

Eastern Massage Therapy:

See Asian Massage Therapy.

Effleurage:

A basic technique of Swedish Massage involving smooth and gliding strokes. The massage therapist uses both hands in this principle stroke of Swedish Massage.

Esalen Massage:

This is a type of massage therapy combining elements of Swedish Massage with sensory awareness principles and environmental sensitivity. It was developed at the Esalen Institute in Big Sur, California.

Fascia:

These are the connective tissues surrounding and supporting the muscles, organs and bones of the body.

Friction:

A basic technique of Swedish Massage. It involves rubbing and deeper penetration of the skin through circular motions of the hands during the massage treatment.

Hot Stone Massage:

This is a popular means of treating specific ailments. It involves placing different-sized heated stones on the affected body parts. Some massage therapists combine hot stone methods with Shiatsu or traditional Asian Massage Therapy (AMT) types. They place the stones according to specific meridians, channels, pressure points, and Chakras.

Ki:

The Japanese form of Chi, the life force or energy.

Kurashova Method:

A form of Russian Medical Message. It involves over 100 types of strokes to address issues of pain and to help athletes recover.

Medical Massage:

Medical Massage is a form of Swedish Massage. Under the prescription of a physician, the practitioner provides the client with specifically medically-directed forms of therapeutic massage.

Meridians:

These are pathways along which the energy or life force flows. They are also known as channels or Chakras.

Myofascial Release:

This technique of massage focuses on the fascia. It employs hands, fingers, elbows, forearms, and palms in smooth, slow, and long strokes to mobilize and stretch the fascia.

Oriental Massage Therapy:

See Asian Massage Therapy.

Petrissage:

This is a basic technique of Swedish Massage. It involves kneading the flesh.

Prana:

The Indian version of the Japanese Ki or Chinese Qi/Chi – life force or energy.

Reflexology:

This type of massage focuses on the zones of the feet and sometimes the hands. The practitioner applies pressure to these zones to free the specific related body parts of pain, anxiety, stress, etc.

Reiki:

Reiki is a hands-off version of massage therapy based on traditional Asian methods of medicine and massage. Using the concepts of Chakras and life forces, Reiki practitioners use their hands to transfer energy to the needed parts and to restore balance.

Rolfing:

The Rolfing Method is a technique aiming to reorganize the body structure through deep manipulation of the myofascial system of the body.

Rosen Method:

This is a system of non-invasive touch and verbal communication. Touch or massage is utilized to detect muscular contraction causing health problems. Verbal expression is used to discover any emotional issues.

Shiatsu:

This is a Japanese form of acupressure. Translated, Shiatsu means "finger pressure." The practitioner applies pressure to specific Ki channels or meridians to restore the balance of energy. Shiatsu rates are high in popularity among Western and Asian cultures as a form of healing therapy.

Sports Massage:

Sports Massage is a variation of Swedish Massage. While Swedish Massage treats the entire body, Sports Massage focuses only on specific parts. It is directed towards maintaining, improving, and rehabilitating the health of athletes. As a result, Sports Massage is subdivided into three categories of treatment: maintenance, event, and rehabilitation. Variations include Equine Sports Massage, designed specifically for racing horses.

Structural Integration:

This term is the original name for Rolfing. It also describes various types of massage therapies and bodywork used to integrate the structure of the body. An example of Structural Integration is Deep Tissue Massage.

Swedish Massage Therapy:

This is the standard and most popular form of Western massage therapy. Its focus is only on the physical healing of the body. It is a traditional form of Western massage therapy. Swedish Massage is the root of many other types of massage, including Deep Tissue Massage, Sports Massage, Medical Massage, and Rolfing. The basic techniques consist of Effleurage, Petrissage, Friction, and Tapotement.

Tapotement:

This is a basic technique of Swedish Massage. It involves using cupped hands, the edge of the hand, or the fingers to stroke gently the client with brief, quick, alternating taps.

Thai Massage:

Is a form of Asian Massage Therapy based upon the principles of Oriental or Eastern Medicine. It involves the manipulation of the client's body together with other techniques. These include acupressure. Thai Massage is often combined with Yoga to create Thai Yoga Massage.

Trigger Point Massage Therapy:

This is a type of massage therapy utilizing the concept of "Trigger Points." Trigger points are centers found usually in muscles that radiate pain to other parts of the body. By pressing the Trigger Points, you reduce pain. Variations of Trigger Point Massage include Bonnie Prudden Myotherapy.

Tui Na:

This is an original form of the Chinese traditional healing system. It relies on the concept of the Qi or Chi life force flowing along meridians or channels. Tui Na or Tuina works with the life force or energy to restore health. It utilizes acupressure, rubbing, pressing, waving, shaking, percussion and manipulation.

Western Massage Therapy:

A term used to describe massage originating in the West and/or demonstrating a focus on or utilization of Western medical theory and practice. In traditional Western massage therapy, the focus is always on the physical body. This differs from Asian or Eastern massage therapy with its holistic approach. Typical forms of Western massage therapies are Swedish Massage, Sports Massage, and Medical Massage.

Zones:

This is the term used in Reflexology to define the points of manipulation used by the practitioner to help the patient regain health, relax and reduce stress. Each zone on the foot or hand corresponds to a central body organ or part.

Don't miss out!

Visit the website below and you can sign up to receive emails whenever Dr. Robertino Bedenian publishes a new book. There's no charge and no obligation.

https://books2read.com/r/B-A-YQGQ-JDBSB

Also by Dr. Robertino Bedenian

Fitness Over 60 For Women – How to Stay Fit And Healthy As You Age

Does Back Pain Go Away? 10 Answers To The Most Acute Back Pain Issues

Massage Bible - A Beginners Guide To Western And Eastern Massage Therapy

Going Vegan - How To Vegan Without Going Crazy

Chiropraktik - Was Steckt Eigentlich Dahinter?

Massagen: Ein Überblick Über Westliche Und Östliche Massagetechniken

Natuerlich Abnehmen, Schlank Und Endlich Fit Sein

P.S. Ich Liebe Dich: Wenn Liebe So Einfach Wäre

Was Tun Bei Rückenschmerzen, Bandscheibenvorfall Und Ischiasschmerzen: 10 Antworten Zu Den Häufigsten Fragen Bei Rückenschmerzen

Was Tun Gegen Schlafapnoe, Schlafstörungen Und Schnarchen

Self-Help Books for Women

Diabetes How to Help: Everything You Need to Know About Diabetes Type 1 and Type 2

Diet and Workout Planner: How to Stay Healthy and Get Fit for Life

Everything I Know About Love

The Sleep Easy Solution Book: How to Stop Sleep Apnea, Snoring, and Sleep Disorders

Your Super Gut Feeling Restored – How to Restore Your Life Energy and Overall Health from The Inside Out

Watch for more at https://booksummarypublishing.com.

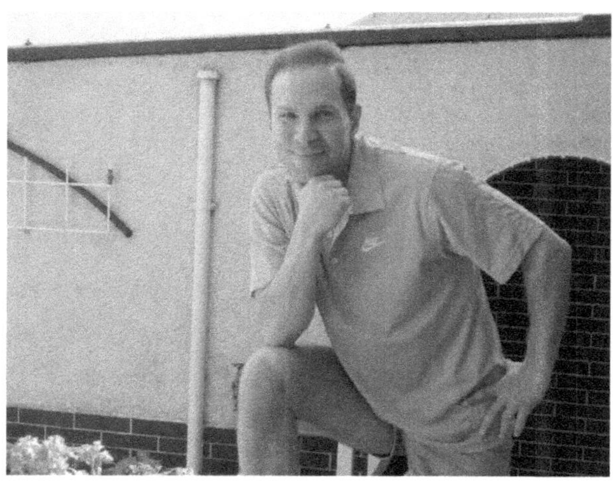

About the Author

Dr. Robertino Bedenian is a qualified fitness instructor accredited by the German Olympic Committee, a health and nutrition expert, and the author of several books on diet, health, and fitness!

For more than twenty years he has been a fitness coach at the sports university teaching aerobics, back gymnastics, stretching, high-intensity interval training (HIIT), power gymnastics, and athletic sports.

On his website, he has published more than 300 articles about the vegan lifestyle covering diet and health recommendations, detoxication programs, fitness guidelines, and disease-related topics. He is part of a family with an orthopedic surgeon, a physical therapist, an osteopath, and an alternative practitioner.

He is also the founder of the brand "**Going Vegan**" selling high-quality supplements for optimal health.

You are more than welcome to check his website for more details: https://goingveganhealthbenefits.com.

His brand has been awarded continuously with 5-star feedback by customers for its outstanding product quality.

Dr. Bedenian is also the founder of the book company "**Book Summary Publishing**" publishing summaries and workbooks of Amazon #1 bestselling non-fiction books.

If you want to learn more about the summaries and workbooks that he has published so far, please visit his website:

https://booksummarypublishing.com

Read more at https://booksummarypublishing.com.